Religious Responses to Pandemics and Crises

W0234700

Religious Responses to Pandemics and Crises explores various dimensions of the interrelations between the individual, community, and religion. With their global scope, the contributions to this volume represent reflections on the rich and multifaceted spectrum of human responses in a variety of different religions and cultures to the current SARS-2-COVID-19 pandemic and similar crises in the past.

The contributions are organized in three thematic parts focusing on strategies, rituals, and past and present responses to pandemics and crises. They reflect on the intersection of personal or communal responses and state-mandated policies relative to SARS-2-COVID-19 while outlining different strategies to cope with the pandemic crisis. Timely questions explored include:

- How do individuals connect with or disconnect from religious and spiritual communities during times of personal and collective crises, including pandemics?
- How do religious practices such as rituals bridge individuals and communities?
- How do religious texts from past and present highlight and represent crises and pandemics?

Dynamic and multidisciplinary in its inquiry, this volume is an outstanding resource for scholars of religion, theology, anthropology, social sciences, ritual theory, sex and gender studies, and contemporary medical science.

Sravana Borkataky-Varma is an Instructional Assistant Professor at the University of Houston, Texas, and a Research Fellow at CSWR, Harvard University.

Christian A. Eberhart is a Professor of Religious Studies at the University of Houston, Texas, USA.

Marianne Bjelland Kartzow is a Professor of New Testament Studies at the University of Oslo, Norway.

Routledge Studies in Religion

Domestic Demons and the Intimate Uncanny
Edited by Thomas G. Kirsch, Kirsten Mahlke and Rijk van Dijk

Jews and Muslims in London and Amsterdam
Conflict and Cooperation, 1990–2020
Sipco J. Vellenga and Gerard A. Wiegers

Alternative Spirituality, Counterculture, and European Rainbow Gatherings
Pachamama, I'm Coming Home
Katri Ratia

Religious Freedom and the Global Regulation of Ayahuasca
Edited by Beatriz Labate and Clancy Cavnar

Interreligious Encounters in Europe
Sites, Materialities and Practices
Edited by Jan Winkler, Laura Haddad, Julia Martínez-Ariño and Giulia Mezzetti

Modern Debates on Prophecy and Prophethood in Islam
Muhammad Iqbal & Said Nursi
Mahsheed Ansari

Religious Responses to the Pandemics and Crises
Isolation, Survival, and #Covidchaos
Edited by Sravana Borkataky-Varma, Christian A. Eberhart, and Marianne Bjelland Kartzow

For more information about this series, please visit: https://www.routledge.com/religion/series/SE0669

Religious Responses to Pandemics and Crises

Isolation, Survival, and #Covidchaos

Edited by
Sravana Borkataky-Varma,
Christian A. Eberhart, and
Marianne Bjelland Kartzow

Routledge
Taylor & Francis Group
LONDON AND NEW YORK

First published 2024
by Routledge
4 Park Square, Milton Park, Abingdon, Oxon OX14 4RN

and by Routledge
605 Third Avenue, New York, NY 10158

Routledge is an imprint of the Taylor & Francis Group, an informa business

British Library Cataloguing-in-Publication Data
A catalogue record for this book is available from the British Library

Library of Congress Cataloging-in-Publication Data
Names: Borkataky-Varma, Sravana, editor. | Eberhart, Christian, editor. | Kartzow, Marianne Bjelland, 1971– editor.
Title: Religious responses to the pandemic and crises : isolation, survival, and #Covidchaos / edited by Sravana Borkataky-Varma, Christian A. Eberhart, and Marianne Bjelland Kartzow.
Description: Abingdon, Oxon ; New York, NY : Routledge, 2024. | Includes bibliographical references and index.
Identifiers: LCCN 2023008047 | ISBN 9781032281223 (hardback) | ISBN 9781032281254 (paperback) | ISBN 9781003295402 (ebook)
Subjects: LCSH: COVID-19 Pandemic, 2020—-Religious aspects—Case studies. | Crisis management—Religious aspects—Case studies.
Classification: LCC RA644.C67 R4584 2024 | DDC 362.1962/4144—dc23/eng/20230527
LC record available at https://lccn.loc.gov/2023008047

ISBN: 978-1-032-28122-3 (hbk)
ISBN: 978-1-032-28125-4 (pbk)
ISBN: 978-1-003-29540-2 (ebk)

DOI: 10.4324/b22930

Contents

Acknowledgments

This edited volume is about human suffering and grief, specifically as the result of the recent COVID-19 pandemic and other similar crises of the past. It is also about how these experiences can lead and have led humans in various religious groups and communities around the globe and throughout history to resilience and new forms of affirmation of life. As such, this book aims at making a positive contribution toward mitigating the pandemic's immediate and imminent consequences.

However, we need to pause for a moment and acknowledge that many people have lost their lives due to the pandemic and/or because of other factors in our societies that may or may not be directly related to this event. Some of these people were beloved family members, some were friends, some were respected colleagues at work, students, the list is long. Some were people we barely knew, and yet their fates touched us. One of these people was Audrey Gale Hall (08/03/2000 – 02/09/2023). A contributor to this very volume, Audrey was a brilliant student and recent graduate of the Religious Studies Program at the University of Houston. As editors, we were deeply saddened to have received the news of her passing and are grieving her loss. May this volume be a lasting testimony in honor and remembrance of her.

Creating a volume like this always involves a multitude of people, some named and some anonymous. Thank you so much! We are grateful to all the contributors from various places, institutions, and contexts around the world. We give thanks to Keith E. McNeal for coining the powerful term "#Coronachaos." This inspired the subtitle of this volume. It is also our privilege to express our gratitude to Ashlin Rae Vance for providing editorial assistance and for compiling the indices. Finally, we are very thankful to the editors and production team in the publishing house for their interest in the topic of this volume and for the smooth cooperation.

Sravana Borkataky-Varma
Christian A. Eberhart
Marianne Bjelland Kartzow

Acknowledgments

Contributors

Soham Al-Suadi is a Professor of New Testament at the University of Rostock, Germany.

Dace Balode is a Professor of Biblical Studies and Dean of the Faculty of Theology at the University of Latvia, Riga, Latvia.

Marianne Bjelland Kartzow is a Professor of New Testament Studies at the Faculty of Theology University of Oslo, Norway.

Sravana Borkataky-Varma is an Instructional Assistant Professor at the University of Houston, Texas, and a Fellow at Harvard University, USA.

Christian A. Eberhart is a Professor of Religious Studies and Director of the Religious Studies Program at the University of Houston, Texas, USA.

Audrey Gale Hall was a recent graduate of the Religious Studies Program at the University of Houston, Texas, USA.

Ma. Maricel S. Ibita is an Associate Professor at the Department of Theology, Ateneo de Manila University, Quezon City, Philippines.

Ma Marilou S. Ibita is an Associate Professor at the Department of Theology and Religious Education, De la Salle University, Manila, Philippines and a visiting professor at the Faculty of Theology and Religious Studies at the Katholieke Universiteit Leuven, Belgium.

Loreen Maseno is a Research Fellow at the Faculty of Theology, University of Pretoria, South Africa.

Keith E. McNeal is an Associate Professor of Anthropology at the University of Houston, Texas, USA, and a Visiting Senior Lecturer at the University of the West Indies – Trinidad & Tobago.

Linards Rozentāls is a Lutheran pastor and lecturer at the University of Latvia, Riga, Latvia.

Dheepa Sundaram is an Assistant Professor of Hindu Studies, Critical Theory and Digital Religion at the University of Denver, USA.

Milo-Rhys K. Teplin di Padilla is an independent researcher.

Ilze Ūdre is a Bachelor of Theology and Religious Studies.

Aaron Michael Ullrey teaches Religious Studies at the University of Houston and is a Sanskrit language instructor at Naropa University, USA.

Elisa Uusimäki is a Professor of Hebrew Bible and Early Judaism at the University of Aarhus, Denmark.

Korinna Zamfir is a Professor of Biblical Studies and Ecumenical Theology at the Faculty of Roman Catholic Theology of the Babeş-Bolyai University of Cluj, Romania.

1 Introduction

Sravana Borkataky-Varma, Christian A. Eberhart and Marianne Bjelland Kartzow

Humans around the entire globe are suffering from the present pandemic situation that has been around for much longer than initially anticipated. Humans are 'social animals.'

In his *Pensées*, Blaise Pascal famously wrote: "Tout le malheur des hommes vient d'une seule chose, qui est de ne savoir pas demeurer en repos, dans une chambre." This translates freely as: "All of humanity's problems stem from one thing that they don't know how to sit quietly in a room alone." Yet one of the most effective measures to cope with the disease is physical distancing (also called 'social distancing'), and for many of us, this just means sitting at home quietly. What does this mean for humans individually and corporately around the globe? This volume focuses on the reality and construction of human identity as communal beings as well as reasons for isolation and distance from others. By visiting different religious groups and communities around the globe, it makes a positive contribution toward mitigating the pandemic's immediate and imminent consequences. It explores the theory and practice of human contact versus distance within the matrix of religion, gender, and ethnicity and in situations of disease and pandemics including the demands on pedagogy. Academic disciplines include comparative religious studies, anthropology, sociology, and psychology.

The following pages first relate personal experiences and impressions of the editors with the pandemic and their responses. This section is followed by an overview of the volume's contents.

1 Sravana Borkataky-Varma's Story

On March 24, 2020, I was sitting at a desk in New Delhi, India, responding to emails. My mother-in-law entered the room with pressing news. India's prime minister, Mr. Narender Modi, ordered a total lockdown, banning all citizens from coming out of their homes. This restriction applied to 1.3 billion people. "Every state, every district, every lane, every village will be under lockdown."[1] The lockdown would begin on March 25, 2020, the very next day.

DOI: 10.4324/b22930-1

I am from India, but my home is in Houston, Texas, in the United States. I return to India often to see my family and conduct research on the larger space of gender and bodies in the Hindu *Śākta* (goddess) tantra. I was visiting my family on that fateful day in New Delhi, and I was scheduled to leave for Houston later that week. Complete chaos ensued, in my house and around the city. I had only a few hours to leave the country, and daily news was already flooded with COVID-19's global spread and shocking death tolls.

I called the travel company that helped me purchase my original ticket and shared the news. On the other end of the phone line, the voice calmly said, "Can you get to the airport in the next three hours?" I said, "Yes!," almost shouting. The kind gentleman secured me a plane ticket.

I reached the International Terminal at New Delhi airport a few hours later. It was mayhem. Hundreds and hundreds of people were trying to get into the terminal; they could speak to airline staff, but the guarded security would not let them enter. Clutching my paperwork, I hoped for the best. After many struggles, I was able to show my changed reservation, and I made my way into the terminal. Some hours later, I was inside an aircraft, and I was headed to Texas.

I left just in time. The all-India, 21-day lockdown in 2020 actually lasted sixty-eight days. It was followed by several phased, partial, and full lockdowns extending into 2021. According to the World Health Organization, in India from "3 January 2020 4:50 pm CET to 6 December 2022, there have been 44,673,783 confirmed cases of COVID-19 with 530,633 deaths."[2] The true number of cases and deaths is likely higher. In urban areas, deaths may have been mislabeled to avoid complex legal complications, and in rural areas, deaths may simply not have been reported to authorities.

Life in Houston was different from India and also different than other places in the United States. Houston never experienced prolonged lockdowns. Grocery shelves, while not full, were never empty. Most stores swiftly pivoted to online ordering and curbside pickup. The independent spirit of Texas was tempered by officials urging the public to take care. As recently as July 2020, a Harris County judge wrote on Twitter, "COVID-19 is rising again in our community, and we need to protect the unvaccinated. Mask up y'all," while the governor urged "personal responsibility rather than government mandates."[3] My family did our part, masking up, social distancing, and volunteering at a vaccination site so that we could be some of the first Texans vaccinated.

First-generation immigrants like me live a dual life. We are not refugees. We made a conscious choice to not live in our birth country. Yet, we are connected to current events of our country of origin; we are personally connected to everything that happens because our families still live there. My family and closest set of friends worried about family and friends back home.

Amidst the worry, our community of immigrants took action. We moved toward cooking meals, sharing recipes, getting tips on how to give a haircut; in short, we experienced a new bond. Friendly Zoom calls, informative emails, and so much social media drew us together. In a way, we were ready for the lockdowns, for we already had habits to communicate with far-off family. The internet had been an international bridge, and now the same technology and tech skills we used to communicate with South Asia could be used to connect in the United States, even to connect in our neighborhoods.

After a few weeks of living with just my family, so-called pandemic bubbles formed; while still isolated, we could at least see select people in person, supported by mutual agreement and trust. Another family and my family started meeting for dinner every Friday, taking turns hosting. We named our group "Friday Meetups," still very much active, more than two and a half years since we first formed the group. We set out the fine china, learned to fold napkins into fancy shapes, and made cocktails with whatever alcohol was available in the local wine store. We dressed up, and we counted our blessings. As a group, our appreciation was focused on the here and now, i.e., focus on today and try not to worry about tomorrow. There was sweetness in being together with a few while isolated from so many, including our families.

This alternate existence was in full swing; yet every morning and every evening, considering the time difference, we called our families and friends in India and Nepal, trying to find ways to navigate and provide support in a very strange time. Communication and support ranged from person to person. Amid all this communication, there was also a flood of religious videos coming through the internet: astrologers making all sorts of predictions, people suggesting dietary changes, mantra healers offering to provide you with a protective shield, the list is long. Some of these videos were forwarded by loved ones through WhatsApp,[4] others were curated for us by social media algorithms. Who would not want a mantra shield, a dietary change to make us immune to COVID-19, or to make sense of the time using planets and stars?

Like most of Generation X, our knowledge of the pandemic came from history books. We lived through the terror of AIDS, but COVID-19 was a different type of pandemic. Diseases were not a ready metaphor in our books, as they had been for the generation before, who read Camus' *The Plague* (1947) or reacted to the consumption in Dostoevsky's *Crime and Punishment* (1866) and Mann's *The Magic Mountain* (1927). We had Marquez's *Love in the time of Cholera* (1985) and we had King's apocalyptic *The Stand* (1978), but the arts and letters had not prepared us for COVID. Our cinema held hope that brave scientists would prevent pandemics, such as in *Outbreak* (1995), little did we know the disease would be as widespread as the one in *The Omega Man* (1971) and its remake *I am Legend* (2007). We braced ourselves for more deaths, even the disintegration of society, and we watched wise scientists befuddled. As a scholar of Hindu traditions, I had some knowledge of diseases in the context of Hindu divinity, but I needed to look deeper.

Unique Hindu responses to the pandemic became apparent. In particular, a picture circulated on social media in which there were two men in masks—one appeared to be a devotee, the other a priest. The priest, wearing a surgical mask, stood, with folded hands, behind a *Śiva liṅgam* (an abstract or aniconic representation of the Hindu god *Śiva*), and the *liṅga* too wore a surgical mask. Such images of deities wearing masks had been used to bring awareness to air pollution in India in 2019. Surgical masks, since the advent of COVID-19, have taken a different significance in human lives across the world. The image was as descriptive as it was prescriptive. Just as humans wear masks, so does the superhuman *Śiva* (this is not out of the ordinary, for *liṅgas* in some temples are daily dressed in clothing). Furthermore, in this image, Śiva is telling the viewer that he or she should wear a mask. The gods in Hinduism are utterly transcendent, but, at the same time, they are immanent in the world; they are affected by the world just as humans are affected. This is not to suggest that Śiva could contract COVID-19, but Śiva wants his followers to be safe and wear masks.[5]

I paused on this image of masked men and a masked god for a while, reading through most of the comments. From then on, my social media algorithm sent me an array of images, including temples live streaming *pūjās* to the goddess Śitalā and also to the novel Corona Devi, a goddess new to the scene but perfectly suited to her current time.[6] I had become a subconscious consumer. These stories and images shaped my understanding, via the algorithms, regardless of whether I actively sought them or not. Strategies for COVID-19 management and protection spread throughout South Asia, reworking a wide range of deities and rituals.[7] Dheepa Sundaram, in her chapter "Pandemic Puja: Corona Devi, Corona Asur, and the Viral Campaign to Reaffirm Analog Ritual Power," explores social media and the power of rituals, demonstrating that new forms of communication can strengthen faith as well as a host of challenges in traditional rituals and deities.

Such developments under COVID-19 duress are not unique or restricted to Hindu traditions. Hardships, historically, propel religiosity and encourage religiousness (Pargament, 2001; Weber, 1920/1993). Booming sales of religious books, including the Bible, were reported in the first weeks of the global pandemic (Coyle, 2020). Increases in prayer were reported in polls globally (Bentzen, 2020; Boguszewski et al., 2020).

Novel and repurposed supernatural entities are not unique to South Asia. Similar to the advent of the Hindu *Coronadevī*, Natalie Lang describes the comeback in 2020 of Saint Corona, previously removed from the Catholic calendar.

> Saint Corona is sometimes depicted with her two deathly palm trees to which she was tied when they were bent down to tear her apart when bouncing up. She became a martyr at the age of 16 for comforting the soldier Victor while he was tortured because of his Christian faith in places ranging from Syria to Italy, depending on the sources, at unknown date around the first to fourth century.[8]

But this saint's return is not without controversy. Elizabeth Harper traces attributions of Corona to be the saint of epidemics to a controversial, right-wing Catholic website. The first instance that I can find of St. Corona getting cited along with "plague," "epidemic," or similar words was on March 11, when Gloria.tv, a right-wing Catholic version of YouTube, posted an article called "There Is a SAINT CORONA and She Is the Patron Saint Against EPIDEMICS."[9]

All these feeds, which I was fast consuming, led me to think deeper about how Hindus have dealt with illnesses and plagues. *Devī Śitalā*, the smallpox goddess, a goddess of skin eruptions, came to mind again. She is found in Sanskrit scriptures and in regular folk depictions across South Asia, astride her donkey, carrying her medicine pot and winnowing fan.[10]

In 2016, while performing research during the sweltering summer heat in Puducherry, *nee* Pondicherri, I engaged a temple priest in a fascinating conversation about the goddess *Śitalā*. I asked the priest about where I could find a *Śitalā* temple, for many books documented several temples to this Goddess in Tamil Nadu, a state in India. The priest looked perplexed. Since smallpox was eradicated, he argued, and since cases of chicken pox and measles are not severe, people do not necessarily seek the protection of the goddess *Śitalā* (folks in Bengal and throughout Northern India may not share this opinion).[11] Furthermore, it is known that worshipping such a goddess is risky, for if the devotee is too invested, she may decide to visit the worshipper, granting a vision that makes the worshipper sick with heated skin eruptions (Stewart, 1995; White, 2003).

We continued to speculate about how some gods and goddesses become popular and others can go out of fashion. In jest, we wondered what would happen if smallpox returned, afflicting people in the current day. Would She also be back in vogue (pun intended)? Our concern with diseases and goddesses may have been prescient. Smallpox has not returned. Corona arrived. As Corona remains with us, so do Corona deities. The best we hope is that *Coronadevī* be pacific and merciful.

Hindu traditions' relationship to diseases, disease-protecting deities, and cures is addressed in Aaron Michael Ullrey's chapter "Diseased Rites: Magic Tantras and Deployed Illness." He argues that magic tantras reveal the means to inflict disease upon an innocent person, but the same sources also reveal remedies, remedies that may even grant superhuman health. Aside from that particular context, a Hindu devotee seeking a cure may engage in a wide spectrum of rituals, prescribed and assisted by priests. Such rituals can range from magic, seeking to alter the world using manipulative ritual actions, to everyday prayers, beseeching mercy, and intervention by a beloved god. Protective and healing powers may be sought in person, in temple spaces, or through direct, physical communication with a cleric, but they can also be sought online.

Returning to a prior statement, through the varied stages of the pandemic, I became a secondary consumer of religious solutions. COVID-19 was everywhere, and it shaped my subconscious mind more than I expected. Realizing the depths of subconscious influence, I needed to write and research to make sense of the pandemic that had altered my professional, social, and family life. This subconscious consumer intake led me to partner with my two colleagues, Christian Eberhart and Marianne Bjelland Kartzow, and the result is the book before you right now.

2 Christian A. Eberhart's Story

My story with COVID-19 has been marked by feelings of loneliness and isolation. For me as a professor at the University of Houston in Texas, the growing epidemic that developed into a pandemic was, in late 2019 and for several months in early 2020, just a news item from remote Asia. Yet suddenly, the first cases of infection and infection-related deaths were reported from Northern Italy, then elsewhere in Europe. Wherever the virus arrived, hospitals were quickly filled with patients who had to be treated in strict isolation. Many of these patients died from severe acute respiratory syndrome. As no medication against the virus was available during the initial months of the pandemic, physical distancing (also called 'social distancing') and wearing face masks were among the first measures that individuals had to follow. Furthermore, governments worldwide ordered lockdowns; shops, schools, and offices closed for a few weeks, then several months. Many other measures followed. There was no precedent of decisions being made so fast and of such a scale in the modern world. Out of compliance with some of these measures, the university where I teach decided to extend its 2020 one-week spring term break by another week, only to resume teaching thereafter in online mode. For more than a year, this became the teaching mode for all academic instructions. Campus life came to a standstill.

All of these measures severely impacted the lives of humans around the globe. I was fortunate. I did not get sick with the virus, and my immediate and extended family did not experience any cases of infection or death cases. Others were not so fortunate. News networks featured interactive online maps that displayed data about the numbers of infected people in countries around the globe and the numbers of those who had died. According to these, countries that had taken protective measures more seriously and implemented them immediately had a significantly lower death toll than others. And yet, I am mourning friends who have attracted COVID-19 and passed away because of it. Estimates of deaths vary between almost 7 million (according to the count of Johns Hopkins University) and anywhere between 16 and 28 million (according to other sources), making COVID-19 one of the deadliest pandemics in history. The threat to everyone's life was real. That was a profound and terrifying experience.

The situation started to change when vaccines against COVID-19 were finally made available in the summer of 2021. I got vaccinated as soon as they were made available, and I have also received booster shots. The pandemic has, ever since then, lost some of its devastating power around the globe, although it still remains a threat to vulnerable populations. What remains for most, however, is an extended experience of isolation and loneliness. A month before the start of the pandemic in the United States, my family and I had just moved to a new home in Houston. The mandatory lockdown implied that we could not even introduce ourselves to our neighbors. It would be months until we dared to knock on their doors to get to know them. And even then, we carefully negotiated how much physical distance we would maintain, that we would wear face masks, and our names were placed on a list for potential tracking should an infection ensue. We followed the rules. All of this shows how much any kind of social life was impacted in those days. During this time, we started weekly Zoom meetings on Saturdays to connect with family members in my native Germany, among other places. Modern communication technology opened doors for regular encounters and exchanges that we had not considered before the pandemic. But it also became clear that such encounters lacked a vital dimension of personal immediacy and could not replace actual physical visits. Yet, international travel was banned for a long time.

These decisions also affected individuals and communities, including religious ones. My church congregation, which belongs to a Lutheran denomination in the United States of America, soon started broadcasting its worship on YouTube. It was only a reduced worship version. Church hymns were chanted by a few paid worship staff members. For the safety of all, sermons and other worship components, including the Eucharistic liturgy, were actually recorded separately and then patched together for streaming on the online platform. The Eucharist as such was made available in the parking lot of the church; people could drive up to the church, and the pastor or other church staff members would distribute bread and wine to them (this is similar to the practice described in the contribution by Ilze Ūdre, Dace Balode, and Linards Rozentāls). After about one year, the church started to offer worship services outdoors. Church members were asked to bring foldable lawn chairs to be set up in one of the parking lots and the adjacent lawn. Families could sit together, but the required physical distance between family groups had to be maintained. One morning, I noticed that a police officer closely supervised the event from a distance, ready to intervene in case of a violation of protocol. The officer did not need to take any action … After several months, things went back to normal; the congregation has, since then, gathered inside the church building as it had done before. The practice of live-streaming the worship was maintained; this is perhaps one collateral benefit of the pandemic experience. A lasting change is that during Eucharist, wine is now poured into an individual cup that every participant receives. Before the pandemic, this was but an option of personal preference; the ritual had generally been celebrated with a common cup that was received by all. The future will show whether this traditional practice will ever be implemented again.

COVID-19 grew into a global pandemic within five months. It made governments worldwide react rapidly to this new threat to their societies. As mentioned above, all of this was unprecedented in the modern world and was to affect individuals and communities, including religious ones.

The COVID-19 pandemic brought with it a profound sense of vulnerability to those who thought that they inhabited parts of the globe that were more sheltered than others. In a way, this experience taught many of us, including me, a lesson about vulnerability and mortality, and with it, the physicality of human existence. In the wake of philosophical writings by René Descartes and Immanuel Kant, the Western tradition has had a strong tendency to conceptualize human existence in a dualistic fashion. According to Descartes, humans are set apart from the rest of the world and thus unique through their capacity to think. The Latin motto *cogito, ergo sum*—"I think, therefore I am" —epitomizes this approach. Not the physicality of their natural bodies but the ability of reasoning and its further development have been determined as the typical characteristic of humans. And according to Kant, humans likewise belong to two realms, namely to nature and to the moral world. As members of the former, they are subject to natural laws that they cannot escape. Humans are independent agents because they are reasonable creatures, and it is through reason that they enjoy freedom. In this way, humanity has been conceptualized independently of and as superior to nature; bodies are only secondary phenomena.[12] These thinking human beings, however, have been challenged by a pandemic that attacks their bodies and reminds them of the limitations of such lofty definitions. The capacity of reasoning is, after all, intrinsically intertwined with the natural realm. Acknowledging our vulnerability and mortality is part of the humility of the homo sapiens to embrace human finitude.[13]

In connection with that, the experience of the pandemic also taught many of us how precious the company of family members, friends, neighbors, work colleagues, students, and other people is. As members of the natural world who have the capacity of reasoning, humans are fundamentally social beings. Their social universe is made up of different other beings. Interaction with them is crucial for the definition of human identity and critical to human development. Celebrations with other humans belong to the fabric of social life in all of its diverse shapes; this also applies to religious communities. As such, celebrations are counter-experiences themselves; they are reminders that loneliness and isolation, even though they are inevitable, are succeeded by manifestations of the presence of others to make human existence once more meaningful. Celebrations are, therefore, also festivals of victory over pain and death. In concluding these personal reflections, I want to specifically acknowledge the resilience of those students at my own university and around the globe who needed to face the problem of isolation and the lack of personal contact with classmates and teachers during semesters of pandemic-related lockdown. The recent celebration of graduation amid those who came to honor them and wish them well on their path into the future became all the more important.

3 Marianne Bjelland Kartzow's Story

The pandemic hit all of us globally at more or less the same time, but still very differently. In this volume, we want to dwell on some of these differences. However, we do not only look at the unfortunate outcomes but also highlight experiences and practices from which we can learn something for the future. Perhaps some of the spontaneous or innovative events that emerged during the pandemic can be continued once it is over, teaching us important things about how to practice religion and be in community with one another.

Those who suffered most during the pandemic were, of course, those who got sick, or died, or lost vital aspects of life, such as home, work, or beloved ones. I was not hit too hard. I live in a country that managed to keep the death numbers low by imposing heavy restrictions that the majority of people followed. Still, for me, the pandemic came with a lot of emotional stress and disturbed my usual focus and rhythm. Social isolation and distancing became a huge challenge in my life, as is the case for most extroverts who gain energy from the presence and time spent around others. I missed the community, my community. I missed the exchange. I missed being among friends and colleagues, going out, being social; theater, restaurants, concerts, and so forth. I missed church, congregation, work, and traveling. I missed airports and sitting alone in a hotel lobby watching strangers pass by, mostly oblivious of who is watching them.

I will mention three examples showing how people around me managed to get me out of the isolation and stress I felt by offering creative activities that contributed to some sense of community.

In Norway, one of the restrictions that was imposed early on was that all cafes, restaurants, and bars were closed. The possibility of visiting others outside one's own cohort became limited; only a few people could meet at the same time. For urban dwellers, this meant that parks or the forests around the city became more popular hangouts. The only problem was the weather; winters are long and cold in this part of the world. In the hardest lockdown periods, a good friend of mine found a creative way out of the situation. She invited me to meet her in downtown Oslo, close to the harbor. She brought warm blankets and an extra wool pullover. She had prepared a fantastic red wine toddy in a thermos and provided snacks. We found a bench with a nice view over the fjord and sat one meter apart. We drank fast and experienced a moment of relief, joy, and fellowship as if the pandemic had never happened. We laughed and talked and got cold, but it was worth it. Her creativity and warmth brought me out of isolation while still following the strict regulations (well, except for the Norwegian law prohibiting alcohol consumption outside in public spaces). Long after we could once again enjoy cafes, we continued to meet at this bench, every now and then, nostalgically drinking the same toddy but sitting a little closer. We had developed a special little ritual: an outdoor bar of our own, with fresh and cold air, a fantastic view, and nice company.

An international colleague who had lived in Oslo for some years taught me something very valuable during the pandemic. She could not visit her relatives back home, as travel was not permitted, and remained isolated in a small flat. She decided to try out one of the few activities that were actually allowed during COVID-19: hiking in the forest. She wanted to do it the Norwegian way, that is, as primitive and "natural" as possible. She got hold of all the necessary equipment and went alone out in the woods, on foot or on a bike, to sleep in a tent or some old cabin she found. I was impressed and excited as she told me about this new experience, since, although I am Norwegian, I had yet to experience the Norwegian ways of hiking. She invited me to come along on one of her expeditions. She brought me into the deepest forest, and I set up my tent at a good distance from hers. We made a fire, watched the sunset, had some tea, and went to bed. The experience was amazing, and I admired her so much for her adventurous energy during the pandemic. Like many others, she turned to nature when everywhere else had closed its doors. Nature remained open and abundant, and around Oslo, it offered enough space to keep the distance. For her, the isolation and frustration did not take her initiative away but gave her the inspiration and opportunity to explore the country she was living in. She invited me into her new world and shared with me a local version of Oslo that I had never seen before. It took a foreigner and a pandemic for me to find the beauty of hiking alone in the Norwegian woods.

For two years, Christmas celebrations had partly been canceled due to COVID-19. That is, the religious community activities were restricted due to the pandemic. Proximity to strangers and chanting meant the extra danger of mass infection. Still, the churches in town found creative ways of navigating the restrictions. Their old, vast buildings provided ample space, although not too many people were allowed to meet indoors at the same time. Instead of inviting churchgoers to shared celebrations, congregations rather opened their churches for a couple of hours on Christmas eve and offered people to come and go, with limitations on how many could be present at the same time. One of the churches close to where I live was open for anyone to come. Clergy read from the Bible every hour, and the church musician played some popular Christmas carols. People walked slowly into the room, lit candles, watched the nativity scene, listened to the readings, and sat down in silence. Chanting was, however, not permitted. Just a few minutes before the church was to be closed and the reading from the Gospel was finished, the musician played one of the most famous and emotional Norwegian Christmas songs, *Deilig er jorden*. It was so beautiful. Suddenly one low voice sang along with the music, and soon everybody stood up and followed. All three verses were sung. People were crying, as always when singing this song, but this time it was different. It was initially not allowed, but it was necessary. That moment made Christmas. It was so moving, so special, and so needed. It was community going against the grain; it was heaven on earth; and it was a true celebration of the light shining in the dark.

I survived the pandemic years due to experiences like these: small glimpses of community, togetherness, and connection, despite all the tragedy, restrictions, isolation, and distancing. Such moments in my everyday life encouraged me to persevere, apart but together. This not only demonstrates humanity's ability to persevere but also reveals the ways in which their creativity and innovation prosper in critical situations. Rather than surrendering to isolation, people take action, involving and engaging with one another. Where community, religion, care, and connection take place, people have the ability to overcome isolation and distancing. Hopefully, we will carry some of the valuable things the pandemic taught us into the future.

4 Contents

The present volume is a collection of experiences, voices, and analyses from a variety of contexts with a strong global perspective. Since the pandemic has inflicted shared experiences, humans benefit from broad and interdisciplinary conversations to articulate their responses. Also, scholars need to participate in this discussion; hence, we, the editors, decided to collaborate on this volume. What becomes clear, however, is that, although we were all in the same boat, it seems like the water treated each of us very differently. When it comes to the concept of "religion," this volume also shows how complex it is to develop clear definitions, in particular when facing the same pandemic. We have tried to highlight some shared analytical approaches, such as theologies, rituals, views on plague, illness, and isolation. By including both contemporary and historical perspectives, ancient texts, recent practices, and digital research, the contributions to this volume challenge us to think both globally and comparatively while going into the depths of some case studies. We end this volume with a compelling call to action on how pedagogy needs to shift because our world shifts as well.

In the first section, *Strategies and Theologies Facing Pandemics*, we start in India, with Dheepa Sundaram's chapter, "Pandemic Pūjā: Corona Devi, Coronasur, and how a Viral Twitter Campaign Affirms Analog Ritual Power." In response to COVID-19, "Coronasur" (a virus as a malevolent force) and "Corona Devi" (a goddess of contagion who combats Corona) have emerged, reprising traditional Hindu notions of "good" defeating "evil." Many Hindus hold the view that virtual sacred spaces must have an analog referent that remains the seat of ritual power. Women in rural villages in Uttar Pradesh, West Bengal, Kerala, Tamil Nadu, and Assam have venerated Corona Devi/ Corona Mai to alleviate the devastating impacts of the virus. These goddesses of contagion have gained popularity and sparked global curiosity through social media, spurring a viral corpus of tweets that spotlight physical temples and analog rituals. Sundaram argues that social media posts on Twitter that popularize rituals to Corona Devi create a digital corpus of posts, which in turn strengthens efforts to reopen material sacred spaces, affirming their value and efficacy in combatting COVID-19 and underscoring the economic implications of India's temple economy.

In the second chapter, we visit Kenya. Loreen Maseno's chapter, "Sitting on a Grave: Female Agency and Resistance During the COVID-19 Pandemic in Chiga Village, Kenya" considers how burials during the COVID-19 pandemic in Kenya initially were conducted hurriedly and securitized by the state. Securitization of COVID-19 includes presenting it as an existential threat requiring urgent measures and justifying alternative actions outside the usually prescribed procedure. Maseno places a sharp focus on the fallout between the state and villagers who wanted to view and give a decent send-off to a deceased musician popularly known as "Jachiga." The chapter gives a feminist reflection on this case in the public domain, where the mother and wife of Jachiga sat on the grave in defiance of a call to exhume the dead after a hurried and securitized state-managed burial in the night. Sitting on the grave is localized and dramatic; her-story that captures the state's inadequacies in addressing current COVID-19 burial-related stalemates and lessons learned.

In the next chapter, called "'He has filled the hungry with good things' (Luke 1:53): Theologizing on the Pandemic, *Pagpupuri,* and Pantries," Ma. Maricel S. Ibita and Ma. Marilou S. Ibita explore the New Testament to reflect on the current pandemic. According to them, collective grief had pervaded the year 2020 because of the multilevel and multi-pronged losses of the COVID-19 pandemic. They explore Mary's Magnificat (Luke 1:53) through the lens of the problem of food insecurity. Moreover, they locate Mary in the context of hunger in 1st-century CE Roman Palestine and relate her experiences to the context of the urban poor women community in the Philippines that takes part in erecting community pantries. Next, they analyze the relationship between hunger, the pandemic, Mary, and Jesus and his meals in the Lukan gospel to highlight the flourishing of community pantries in the Philippines. This is finally related to the United Nations Sustainable Goal of Zero Hunger (UNSDG#2).

The second section, *Rituals in Times of Trouble*, employs ritual as a key concept to address religion and crises, pandemics, and the current pandemic. We start with Aaron Michael Ullrey's chapter "Diseased Rites: Magic Tantras and Inflicted Illness." In South Asia, according to him, and especially in the Hindu traditions, diseases are typically depicted as deities and disorders. But in the magic tantras, a disease can be an affliction cast by a human ritualist upon a victim. A knowing sorcerer can deploy disease as a weapon. Magical rituals spread illness as quickly as any contagion, fueled by the hatred and jealousy of the ritualist for his/her client. This chapter highlights ritually inflicting disease in magic tantras belonging to Hindu Śaivism. The *Uḍḍīśatantra*, a generally Śaiva source, and related texts in the so-called Uḍḍ-corpus contain mantras and rituals to inflict and remove a range of disease deities, but sources also present antidotes that confer supernatural health and vigor. Overlap with witchcraft lore and medicine, as well as Ayurveda, is noted throughout. In a discourse dominated by maliciously casting disease upon the unsuspecting, a glimpse of positivity is found.

The next chapter presents a case study from Latvia. Ilze Ūdre, Dace Balode, and Linards Rozentāls ask, "'Can a virus destroy the sacred?' The Latvian

Experience of Holy Communion During COVID-19." This chapter reflects on the experience of Holy Communion during COVID-19 in the Latvian Lutheran congregations, based on the qualitative research conducted in the congregations of the Evangelical Lutheran Church of Latvia (ELCL) and the author's observations in the Latvian Lutheran congregations. The COVID-19 pandemic has affected Holy Communion and the liturgy of church services on a temporary and more permanent level in Latvian Lutheran churches. All surveyed parishes adjusted to the regulations, and there was no particular resistance to the new rules. The restrictions hit more parishes smaller in number, which ceased to celebrate Holy Communion. In the ELCL, there was no serious discussion about celebrating the Eucharist remotely, most likely because of the very high theology of Communion. Communicants in the parishes preferred the individual Eucharist to that of intinction, demonstrating the theological emphasis on vertical communion during Holy Communion. However, this time it highlighted differences between churches that employed advanced digital tools and those that did not.

The topic of Eucharist is also central to the next chapter, which presents historical and contemporary perspectives. The focus is on Romania; after years of the pandemic, the country became the closest neighbor of a tragic new war in Europe. In "Reinvention and the Celebration of the Eucharist in Times of Crises: Biblical and Contemporary Perspectives," Korinna Zamfir takes this point of departure. During crises, both Judaism and emerging Christianity have adapted worship to changed circumstances through a process of ritual transference. The significance of no longer accessible rites and sacred spaces was transferred to new rites and spaces. This led to the invention of the Passover *Seder* following the destruction of the Second Temple and of the early Eucharistic meal after the death of the founding figure. In the process, remembrance enabled a spiritual, virtual communion with foundational events, overcoming temporal and spatial distance. These developments may inform attempts to cope with contemporary crises (pandemics, wars) that prevent access to sacred space and the customary performance of worship. One such solution is the virtual celebration of the Eucharist via narrowcasting platforms allowing real-time, interactive participation. This requires a new understanding of sacred space and the emergence of a theological concept of sacred virtuality. Sacred virtuality involves the conviction that divine power (*virtus*) remains effective in digital environments, transcending physical distance in ways comparable to the ability of remembrance to allow sharing of past foundational events.

The final chapter in this section employs ritual theory to reflect on isolation and community in New Testament letters. Soham Al-Suadi's chapter "Isolation, Community, and Religious Identification: The Ritual World of Early Christian Imprisonment Letters" proposes a detailed reading of some of these biblical texts. In the New Testament, according to her, the tension between isolation and community is particularly evident in religious contexts. Lifestyles and communities are questioned by crisis experiences, re-evaluated, and experimentally implemented. Important experiences that serve the purpose of reorientation are expressed in rituals. This chapter is devoted to the ritual aspects of the early Christian imprisonment letters to the Ephesians, Philippians, Colossians, and Philemon that are all part of the Pauline discourse. They are religious texts that convey accounts of this world and the world to come, as well as death and resurrection, through ritual experiences. Personal and collective experiences of crisis are manifested in rituals and serve religious identification.

In the third section, entitled *Plagues, Infections, and Witchcraft*, we stay in the Bible but move to the Hebrew Bible/Old Testament. Elisa Uusimäki's chapter "Plagues, Withdrawal, and Wayfaring in the Hebrew Bible" investigates the interplay between plagues and (im)mobility in Hebrew Bible texts, which depict plagues as both prompting and inhibiting movement. While plagues are imagined to cause moments of disruption, thus creating anxiety and horror, the texts also attest to practical management strategies and resilience. The analysis falls into two parts. First, Uusimäki explores the plague motif in two narratives in which plagues cause welcome disruptions, enabling the release of Hebrews who find themselves stuck in oppressive or otherwise undesirable situations. The narratives are shown to focus on how YHWH, the puppet master, uses plagues to control things. Second, she analyzes the evidence of legal, narrative, and liturgical texts on detachment from other people. Priestly laws as well as two narratives on kings suggest that a person hit by a plague should withdraw and isolate. In these texts, the focus is on how to handle a threatening plague. Liturgical poetry adds to this picture by elaborating on experiences of loneliness and longing caused by illness-related seclusion, thus drawing attention to how it feels to be hit by a plague.

Audrey Gale Hall's chapter, "The Leper as Transcestor," positions the biblical figure of the leper analogously with transgender people of faith in the United States. This contribution grounds transgender practices of ancestor (transcestor) veneration in the chaos of the Israelite community's rejection of their own relatives in Numbers (*B^{e}midbar*). Those with skin conditions known as *tsara'at* were expelled alongside others whose bodies bore the signs of recent sexual and reproductive functions, which begs the question of how transgender people can religiously respond to their ostracization from faith communities that simultaneously target birthing and promiscuous individuals. The deleterious community health effects of religious rejection and abuse on trans individuals mirror the health impact of untreated leprosy, as does the crisis of houselessness in leprous and transgender populations. By placing the geographic, social, and spiritual position of the leper in conversation with the large-scale exit of transgender people from mainstream American religious life, Hall brings new meaning to Sylvia Rivera's phrase "Queens in Exile."

Milo Rhys K. Teplin di Padilla's chapter, "Constructing the Sacred Self: 21st Century Paganism, Self-Care, and Ascetic Witchcraft," looks at isolation and explores virtual tools as a solution. According to Teplin di Padilla, the isolation measures experienced by practicing pagans during the COVID-19 pandemic allowed for a general assessment of the community at large as well as personal growth in individual practice. By contrasting the different approaches to their faith online, members of this community had to create new means not only of where and how to enact rituals but also how to define sacred space and how they personally related to these terms on a practical and spiritual level. Common practices ranged from Jungian introspective meditation to co-opting mundane domestic tasks as a meditative activity for ritual and prayer. Bonds with other members of similar faiths were almost entirely virtual and allowed for the community to come together as a whole to assess stances on doctrine, social issues, and technological impact on practice.

The last chapter in this volume is "Pedagogy of Death in the Era of #Coronachaos" by Keith E. McNeal. His text reflects upon the experience of teaching a new course on the Anthropology of Death and Mortuary Ritual in the Fall of 2020, commencing six months into the pandemic yet planned before any sign of COVID-19. He adapted the course to teaching online under the excruciatingly complex conditions imposed by the pandemic. COVID-19 then took his grandmother, which he shared by anthropologizing his family's experience as a case study. His students pursued a host of fascinating and revelatory research projects on death and mortuary ritual during the local pandemic. He considers his own pandemic-prompted spirituality as well as the poignant irony of finding more community with his students online than with his family living in another state. Contemplating death and mortuary ritual together in the midst of #Coronachaos was not only pedagogically richer but also a source of solidarity for everyone. He concludes by querying death's deeper history and possible futures in light of COVID-19 as an Anthropocenic disease, a tiny piece of inert RNA that became a global monster.

Notes

1 https://www.nytimes.com/2020/03/24/world/asia/india-coronavirus-lockdown.html. Downloaded on 12/6/2022, at 1:25 PM.
2 https://covid19.who.int/region/searo/country/in. Downloaded on 12/6/200, at 1:48 PM.
3 https://www.houstoniamag.com/health-and-wellness/what-to-know-about-houston-coronavirus
4 WhatsApp is a messaging system which blends short messaging service (SMS) and social networking.
5 Arumugam, Indira. "Do the Gods Have COVID-19 Too?: Protecting Idols, Cherishing Deities," https://ari.nus.edu.sg/20331-44/.
6 Gods and goddesses arising or shifting from minor prevalence to widespread worship has been documented elsewhere in 20th century Hinduisms. Saṃtoṣī Mātā (known as Santoshi Ma) shifted from a minor local deity to a widespread goddess worshipped for prosperity and health by women throughout India and in the

diaspora; her spread was fascilitated by a popular film. Lutgendorf, Philip. "Is There an Indian Way of Filmmaking?" *International Journal of Hindu Studies* 10, no. 3 (2006): 227–256. Das, Veena. "The Mythological Film and Its Framework of Meaning: An Analysis of 'Jai Santoshi Ma'," *India International Centre Quarterly* 8, no. 1 (1981): 43–56.

7 De Siliva, Premakumara, "The Cult of Goddess Pattini at a Time of Pandemic: Gammaduwa as a Strategy of Supernatural Protection," https://ari.nus.edu.sg/20331-91/.

8 Lang, Natalie, "Saint Corona, CoronAsur, and Corona Devi: New Embodiments of the Relationship between Religion and Disease," (blog) *CoronAsur Research Blog*, Accessed December 8, 2022, 1.30 PM, https://ari.nus.edu.sg/20331-25/.

9 Harper, Wlizabeth, "Is St. Corona Really the Patron Saint of Plagues?," Accessed December 8, 2022, 4.28 PM, https://slate.com/human-interest/2020/03/saint-corona-patron-saint-of-plagues.html.

10 Nicholas, Ralph W, "The Goddess Śītalā and Epidemic Smallpox in Bengal," *The Journal of Asian Studies* 41, no. 1 (1981): 21–44. Wadley, Susan S, "Śītalā: The Cool One." *Asian Folklore Studies* 39, no. 1 (1980): 33–62.

11 Dasgupta, Deepsikha, "New Diseases, Old Deities: Revisiting Sitala Maa during COVID-19 Pandemic in Bengal," https://ari.nus.edu.sg/20331-75/.

12 Cf. Erbele-Küster/Küster/Roth, *Theologie infiziert*, 31.

13 On the topic of vulnerability, see Brown, "TEDxHouston, The Power of Vulnerability."

Bibliography

Arumugam, Indira, " Do the Gods Have COVID-19 Too?: Protecting Idols, Cherishing Deities," National University of Singapore, Asia Research Institute, https://ari.nus.edu.sg/20331-44/.

Brown, Brené, "TEDxHouston, The Power of Vulnerability," *TED* June 1, 2010, Accessed December 18, 2022, https://www.ted.com/talks/brene_brown_the_power_of_vulnerability/comments.

Das, Veena. "The Mythological Film and Its Framework of Meaning: An Analysis of 'Jai Santoshi Ma'," *India International Centre Quarterly* 8, no. 1 (1981): 43–56.

Dasgupta, Deepsikha, "New Diseases, Old Deities: Revisiting Sitala Maa during COVID-19 Pandemic in Bengal," National University of Singapore, Asia Research Institute, https://ari.nus.edu.sg/20331-75/.

de Siliva, Premakumara, "The Cult of Goddess Pattini at a time of Pandemic: Gammaduwa as a Strategy of Supernatural Protection," National University of Singapore, Asia Research Institute, https://ari.nus.edu.sg/20331-91/

Erbele-Küster, Dorothea/Küster, Volker/Roth, Michael, *Theologie infiziert: Religiöse Rede im Kontext der Pandemie* (Theologische Interventionen 7), Stuttgart: Kohlhammer, 2021.

Gettleman, Jeffrey and Kai Schultz, "Modi Orders 3-Week Total Lockdown for All 1.3 Billion Indians," *New York Times*, https://www.nytimes.com/2020/03/24/world/asia/india-coronavirus-lockdown.html.

Harper, Wlizabeth, "Is St. Corona Really the Patron Saint of Plagues?," Accessed December 8, 2022, 4.28 PM, https://slate.com/human-interest/2020/03/saint-corona-patron-saint-of-plagues.html

Lang, Natalie, "Saint Corona, CoronAsur, and Corona Devi: New Embodiments of the Relationship between Religion and Disease," (blog) *CoronAsur Research Blog*, Accessed December 8, 2022, 1.30 PM, https://ari.nus.edu.sg/20331-25/.

Lutgendorf, Philip, "Is There an Indian Way of Filmmaking?," *International Journal of Hindu Studies* 10, no. 3 (2006): 227–256.

Nicholas, Ralph W, "The Goddess Śītalā and Epidemic Smallpox in Bengal," *The Journal of Asian Studies* 41, no. 1 (1981): 21–44.

Wadley, Susan S, "Śītalā: The Cool One," *Asian Folklore Studies* 39, no. 1 (1980): 33–62.

Wray, Dianna and Catherine Wendlandt, "Here's What You Need to Know about the Coronavirus in Houston," *Houstonia*, https://www.houstoniamag.com/health-and-wellness/what-to-know-about-houston-coronavirus.

Part I

Strategies and Theologies Facing Pandemics

2 Pandemic Pūjā

Corona Devi, Coronasur, and How a Viral Twitter Campaign Affirms Analog Ritual Power

Dheepa Sundaram

Summary and Next Steps

The phenomenon of deifying diseases through figures such as Corona Devi/Corona Mai and Coronasur is an integral part of Hindu teleology. Since this essay would be only the third paper on the Corona Devi/Corona Mai and Coronasur, the topic is ripe for further exploration. Future research should consider how worship of these deities impacts and shapes adherent communities, particularly in Tamil Nadu, where two temples have installed an icon of the goddess. While this study focuses on hashtags and mentions, more analysis of networks of influence and meaning-making within social media would provide valuable insight into how an emerging deity can create virtual devotional publics. For example, further analysis of how temples and priests use Facebook to connect with devotional communities in the context of Facebook's marketing algorithm could show how temple economies rely on cultures of connectivity (Van Dijck 2013) to be economically viable. Additionally, it would be valuable to examine how these divine figures are configured and leveraged within discourses of gender, caste, and class marginalization in India.

1 Introduction

Social media research on religion has been concerned with issues of authority and the role of materiality in digital venues (Cheong 2014; Hoover 2016) and the impact of online religious rhetoric on offline religious engagement (Åhman and Thorén 2021; Young 2004). While Pauline Cheong spotlights how church leaders have used social media platforms to drive engagement with scripture and church attendance, Stewart Hoover's work shows the impact of online spaces in constructing religious authority and materiality of canon. Growing scholarship on these questions shows the complex interactions between digital and analog spaces and how materiality is mediated and reconfigured (Evolvi 2020). Recent studies on digital materiality have explored how material objects are embedded within virtual applications (Evolvi 2020); recordings of religious services can activate or produce a "sensorial experience" (Meyer 2008), and software can function as a material

DOI: 10.4324/b22930-3

object (Hutchings and Mckenzie 2016). Guilia Evolvi notes that in each of these cases, "virtual and tangible characteristics coexist" (Evolvi 2020, 2). While material culture approaches to the study of religion in virtual spaces are growing, most do not yet address whether virtual engagements and communications can drive offline religious engagement (Evolvi 2020). Some of the questions I address here are:

1 How does social media reaffirm the value and efficacy of offline rituals and physical places of worship?
2 What does this tell us about the production of religious authority and the liminality between offline sacred space and digital networks?

Many studies of digital media and religion have considered the concept of "third space"[1] (Hoover and Echchaibi 2014) that focuses on how "digital and social media hail their practitioners into new subjectivities" (Hoover 2016, 17). Stewart Hoover suggests that religious authority in digital spaces is not transferred or recreated but rather co-constituted through the interplay between online and offline. My intervention builds on what he describes as the "conceptual turns" of religious authority within digital media spaces to consider these spaces "anthropologically: in terms of what conceptual and physical geographies they imply and what sorts of cultural meanings and strategies they invoke" (Hoover 2016, 18). The affordances digital spaces provided for religious practices during the COVID-19 pandemic were invaluable, but they did not necessarily convert adherents into digital worshippers. By examining the emergence of Corona Devi[2]/Corona Mai within the Twittersphere in terms of the "physical geographies they imply," we see how the performativity and practices of digital space reaffirm the cultural meaning and authority of the physical sacred. Specifically, as the phenomenon of Corona Devi/Corona Mai went viral, more adherents turned to analog rituals and places of worship for recourse from the virus. Such a turn also reflected the belief that if the goddess could be pacified, then both physical and economic well-being in the form of reopening would follow.

The COVID-19 pandemic has defined all aspects of human life globally for the past three years, and religion and spirituality are no exception. Before the pandemic, 71% of Indians claimed to visit "religious sites or places of worship" at least once a month, while 60% say they pray daily (Sahgal et al. 2021). As access to the analog/physical[3] sacred spaces was restricted, particularly in the first year of the pandemic, virtual means of worship became more prevalent. Virtual prayer services, temple attendance, the emergence of social media religion/spiritual communities, digital ritual services, and other modes of worship unmoored and unconstrained COVID-19 restrictions on physical spaces become prevalent. In Hindu contexts, the response to COVID-19 pandemic includes the emergence of "Corona Devi" (the goddess associated with coronavirus) and "Coronasur" (the virus as a malevolent force), reprising traditional Hindu notions of "good" defeating "evil" (Srinivas 2020). An effigy of Coronasur[4] was burned during a Holi festival in Mumbai in March 2020 representing a ritual destruction of the virus (Lang 2020). Following the imagery of malevolent figures in Brahmanical Hindu mythology (e.g., Śūrpanakhā, Hiraṇyākṣa, and Mahīṣāsura), the effigy was green (to indicate dark skin) with a protruding tongue, sharp long fingernails, large animal-like teeth, horns, and was wearing a garland of red cylindrical objects that represented the COVID-19 molecules (Yadav 2022). Perhaps even more significantly, the effigy held "a board with the text, *ārthikmandī*, meaning 'economic recession'" (Yadav 2022). This speaks to the dual concerns regarding both spiritual and economic health stemming from the COVID-19 pandemic. As Megha Yadav notes, the demonic figure of Coronasur becomes the source of economic troubles rather than government policy (Yadav 2020). Furthermore, such actions show why rituals to Corona Devi hold both spiritual and economic significance.

Throughout the pandemic, Hindu priests have continued to perform rituals in temples, arguing that Corona Devi's (goddess) power can only be "activated" through such practices (Mitra 2020). Since many Hindu priests and adherents assert that virtual sacred spaces and practices must have an analog referent for authority and efficacy, online gatherings and social media engagement can only be partially effective. These context-specific divine figures have gained popularity and sparked global curiosity through social media, spurring a virtual campaign for reopening temples rather than fostering a virtual religious community. Social media (Twitter particularly) popularize figures like Corona Devi and Coronasur to create a virtual corpus of posts that reaffirm the value and efficacy of physical sacred spaces for combating COVID-19. This study will focus on Twitter since it functions as a microblogging digital public square in which media can be shared from multiple sources, but which becomes searchable through hashtags, making the volume of posts as important as the connective functions such as liking, retweeting, and following.

This essay argues that the volume of posts on Twitter which feature rituals for Corona Devi/Corona Mai demonstrate the continued belief in the value and efficacy of analog rituals. The installation of Corona Devi in temples, as witnessed in Tamil Nadu and Kerala, shows how the reopening of Hindu temples and shrines was seen as essential to combat the virus and the economic downturn resulting from the lockdown. These religious arguments for reopening temples buttress the economic concerns surrounding a prolonged lockdown, particularly for the profitable religion industry in India. Such arguments are a stark contrast to those heard in the US that suggested maintaining access to physical places of worship amounts to an issue of "religious freedom." In other words, this virtual network of posts about Corona Devi/Corona Mai rituals reiterates the importance and impact of the material sacred space of the temple as locus of community spiritual health and economic well-being.

This chapter is organized as follows: theoretical foundations which shape online discourse and its impact on offline religious practices (Cheong 2014; Zeiler 2020; Van Dijck 2013); methodology for analyzing tweets and hashtags on Twitter; an overview of the authority of physical sacred space in Hindu contexts; a brief history of disease goddesses and their importance during pandemics; a discussion of the Twitter posts of media showing Corona Devi/Corona Mai *pūjā* (personal worship); and concluding remarks which discuss how the virtual corpus of tweets about Corona Devi/Corona Mai reinforces the importance of analog sacred space as both spiritually and economically beneficial.

2 Theoretical Foundations

Since this essay focuses on the relationship between social media posts and the analog practices and policies that these posts reaffirm, the evidence largely stems from tweets and retweets as well as comments and reactions, which show how these tweets both shape online discourse and point adherents toward physical sacred spaces and practices. I build my work on social media historiography, the use of social media platforms to impact offline religious practices, the question of how virtual religious communities are imbricated into economies, and the efficacy of traditional analog worship spaces and practices. Jose van Dijck argues that social media utilize connecting and sharing functions such as "likes," "shares," and "retweets" to operate as cultural capital; she demonstrates how social media platforms such as Facebook and Twitter are invested in creating networks of capital (Van Dijck 2013). While my argument rests on the volume of tweets by individual users, the principle of connectivity Van Dijck outlines shows how social media can produce a semiotic network through hashtags even when individual posts are not widely shared. Twitter fills gaps that Facebook leaves by providing users the opportunity to participate in broad conversations without "friending" everyone involved. In this sense, it becomes "a tool for connecting individuals and communities of users—a platform that empowers citizens to voice opinions and emotions, that helps stage public dialogues, and supports groups or ideas to garner attention" (Van Dijck 2013, 73). Such connections are reciprocal rather than unidirectional and help facilitate a conversation between digital and analog communities. In this case, we see traditional media outlets covering a phenomenon that gains notoriety in the digital space and subsequently impacts offline religious practices.

In addition to the interplay between communities in physical and virtual spaces, Twitter transforms the relationship between faith-based institutions, religious leaders, and religious adherents. Although earlier characterizations of social media platforms suggest they subvert or disrupt the authority of religious institutions, a growing body of recent scholarship has found "synergetic relationships between online and offline faith beliefs and infrastructures, including how religious leaders shape, sustain, and are being sustained by their latest digital and social media practices" (Cheong 2014, 4). Within Hindu contexts, physical sacred space and material religious figurines remain essential to the efficacy of rituals. In this sense, within the sphere of "digital Hinduism," social media networks and individual actors within these networks are connected intimately to analog religious practices and places of worship (Zeiler 2020). Building on these models, my essay shows how social media functions (like those on Twitter) use digital networks of likes, shares, and retweets to both reiterate and challenge orthodox formulations of religious practice while reinforcing the importance of physical sacred space and practices.

3 Methodology

This research takes a qualitative approach to cataloging tweets, mentions, and retweets with the terms "CoronaDevi," "CoronaMai," and "Coronasur." I examine how tweets that mention rituals to Corona Devi/Corona Mai/Durgā/Coronasur produce a virtual corpus. In turn, this corpus supports policy and legislative actions in India that preserve physical access to temples and shrines during the pandemic.[5] I also explore media reports detailing how temples articulate the need for analog sacred spaces as a bulwark against disease, focusing on the Kāmātcipuṟam Ādhīnam temple complex in Coimbatore, Tamil Nadu that installs "Corona Devi" in May 2021. This complex already includes the Plague Māriyammaṉ[6] temple consecrated nearly one hundred years earlier.

My analysis of Corona Devi focuses on Twitter and catalogs the use of the following hashtags: #CoronaDevi, #CoronaMai, #CoronAsur (and the variations in capitalization) and analogous searches of these terms in posts. I focus on Twitter since the circulation of these terms on Facebook and Instagram did not have the same volume of representation. I have limited my search to January 1, 2020, through June 30, 2021, which corresponds to both when these figures gained popularity and the height of the COVID-19 pandemic in India. Using Twitter's advanced search feature, my purpose is not to show the volume of tweets, although such an analysis also could be useful. Rather, through a selection of tweets and comments, I show how the online compendium of tweets, likes, retweets, and comments points to the importance of the analog sacred space. Nearly every tweet centers on the offline temple that installed Corona Devi and other analog rituals to Corona Devi in rural villages of states such as Tamil Nadu, Kerala, and West Bengal. I also discuss the Durgā *pūjā paṇḍāls* in Calcutta in October 2021, which reconfigure Durgā as Corona Devi and characterize Mahīṣāsura as Coronasur to show how the goddess is superimposed onto traditional Hindu rituals that depict the victory of "good" over "evil." In this sense, each of these examples shows how the Twitterverse, even during the heart of the COVID-19 pandemic, reaffirms the vitality, authority, and efficacy of analog sacred spaces, rituals, and artifacts.

Additionally, nearly every tweet appears to be from an online observer of the rituals, a journalist, or a citizen who engages with media reports about the rituals rather than those who perform the ritual themselves or witness them live.[7] This points to an issue beyond the scope of this essay regarding whose voices are being amplified and in what ways. The rural, caste-oppressed communities that initially perform these rites, those creating *paṇḍāls* for Durgā *pūjā* that picture the goddess in a doctor's coat slaying the virus (Chowdhury 2020) and, the Brahmanical priests in Kāmātcipuṟam Ādhīnam temple Maṭh are not tweeting these rituals or discussing them in virtual platforms. However, pictures of the *paṇḍāl*s with this image of Durgā were shared 71,000 times with over 8,000 reactions on Facebook and subsequently Twitter (Chowdhury 2020). Thus, media reports that often include interviews, photos, and videos, photos by individuals, and artistic renderings such as the viral drawing of Corona Devi pictured in a mask and carrying hand sanitizer (Srinivas 2020) are being shared by individual users on social media. In this sense, while those practicing the rituals may not be avid social media users, their actions have become a part of social media networks.

4 Authority of Physical Sacred Space

In many religious traditions, the analog or physical sacred space as a "gold standard" for worship remains paramount. A vast body of cited scholarship on Hinduism emphasizes the authority of physical sacred space for karmic efficacy (Eck 1982; Granoff and Shinohara 2007; Hudson 2008). Stories of the land express how particular deities can exercise their power. Moreover, every temple requires a *purāṇa,* or story, that explains why this deity should be worshipped in this location and their connection to this place. Digital media has troubled the relationship between the analog sacred space and the ability to access its benefits (Dudrah et al. 2012). Sites like vmandir.com that allow adherents access to *darśan*, or sacred vision and experience of the deity, upon entering the homepage, no longer adhere to the notion that the physical confines of the temple are necessary for divine blessing. Similarly, ritual websites that broker access to temple rituals complicate these boundaries between physical sacred space and the virtual world. Sites such as shubhpuja.co.in or epuja.co.in offer adherents the chance to "book" rituals which are performed in a physical sacred space and receive *prasāda* (food blessed by the deity) all through an online portal. Whether such digital rituals are seen as efficacious remains an open question.

Indeed, when discussing the impact of the COVID-19 pandemic on worship practices, one priest argued that the "closure of temples and shrines has widened the distance between gods and devotees, and the separation cannot be erased through prayers at home" (Press Trust of India 2020). Such an argument is reinforced when women in villages in several regions of India began conducting rituals and chanting mantras to "Corona Mai" in, for example, West Bengal and then later in Uttar Pradesh, Kerala, Assam, and Bihar as an alternative to seeking assistance from hospitals who seemed helpless in the face of the virus (Samanta 2020). The desire to avoid hospitals was in part an expression of distrust of the public healthcare system, particularly by the poor (Samanta 2020), as well as a belief that only the goddess could protect them from harm (Roychowdhury 2020). Some priests said that prayers to the goddess would protect and assist healthcare workers, such as a Kerala priest who created a makeshift idol to Corona Devi in his home and began offering daily prayers (Roychowdhury 2020).

Interviews I conducted with three *dīkṣatar*-s[8] (brahman priests) in Chennai and Bangalore underscore how religious authorities view sacred physical spaces as necessary to achieve karmic goals. They are considered relevant to maintain dharmic responsibilities that would move an adherent toward spiritual goals such as *mokṣa* (liberation) from *saṃsāra* (cycle of rebirth) (Diksatar 2018). Specifically, Mahadeva Diksatar stated, in my conversation with him, that *phalam* (fruit/results) was only possible in *karmabhūmi*[9] (the physical land space of India), where rituals would have efficacy (Diksatar 2018). However, he did note that adherents that conduct rituals through virtual means or by proxy could maintain their dharmic position without moving "up or down," but that such actions would be for *manas* (heart) or *tripti* (satisfaction) (Diksatar 2018). In other words, while conducting worship and rituals outside of analog sacred spaces could not move forward the goal of *mokṣa*, one could maintain ones' spiritual position in the next birth.

During the height of the COVID-19 pandemic, several religious communities found solace in virtual networks, services, and rituals. Virtual *satsangs* (prayer gatherings), video *pūjā*, as well as emerging forms of sacred connection such as virtual reality access to temples, became popular (Mitra 2020). Indeed, VR Devotee and Parampara.app, two applications which sought to bring traditionally analog sacred experiences to adherents through virtual means, may have inadvertently questioned the necessity of physical, offline spaces for ritual efficacy. Though Kalpnik Technologies launched VR Devotee in 2017, its popularity grew during the COVID-19 pandemic. The application offers user-devotees access to an immersive experience of live and recorded temple rituals through a smartphone (Sundaram 2021). Parampara.app is a website that instructs user-devotees how to convert a home into a temple and perform rituals that would conventionally require a priest. This application specifically caters to Tamil Brahmin users evidenced within the interface that asks users to choose between "Iyer, Iyengar, or Madhwa" (three categories of Tamil Brahmins). While Parampara.app was created for the pandemic as a stop-gap measure for Tamil Brahmins who lacked access to priests during the lockdown, VR Devotee sought to increase access to temples more broadly and saw a rise in membership during the first two years of the pandemic (Sundaram 2021). While increasing access to rituals, albeit for different communities, digital applications like Parampara and VR Devotee push the boundaries of how a ritual is conducted, where it is performed, and what constitutes an authentic experience (Sundaram 2021). Each of these applications offers products that question the superior efficacy and authority of physical, offline sacred space. However, neither application has remained as popular since lockdowns have been lifted, indicating that Hindu adherents are not ready to jettison physical sacred space if it is accessible.[10]

5 Who Is "Corona Devi"? The History of Disease Goddesses

During the COVID-19 pandemic, the concern around closing physical temples was palpable. For example, several priests at the Srī Venkateśvara Vāri temple in Tirumala (Tirupati) insisted on keeping the temple open and continuing to conduct rituals to ensure that they were doing everything possible to combat the virus (Press Trust of India 2020). The belief was that "Coronavirus is an *asur* (malevolent divine being) and it can only be killed by divine forces [and that] divinity would rescue devotees from the coronavirus after joint prayers" (Press Trust of India 2020). After the initial wave of the virus, when temples reopened with strict COVID-19 mitigation protocols, some insisted on holding large events such as the Kumbha Mela. Some large religious gatherings did proceed as spiritual beliefs trumped concerns about safety. As one priest who encouraged people to attend the Mela stated, "We are sure the faith in God will overcome the fear of the virus" (Slater and Masih 2021). He later contracted the virus and died (Slater and Masih 2021). When temples were closed between March and May 2020, many Hindu adherents began conducting rituals to Corona Devi, at first in rural locales (Samanta 2020). These rituals were seen as the only available solution to those who had little faith in healthcare providers or facilities (Samanta 2020).

However, the belief that a goddess could remedy what had so far stumped doctors and healthcare providers was rooted in Hindu belief. Corona Devi hails a long tradition of so-called disease goddesses within the Hindu tradition (Srinivas 2020). Historically, disease goddesses have been seen as both the arbiters of disease and sometimes violence and having the ability to protect adherents from such calamities (Samuel 2008, 249; Srinivas 2020). One of the earliest examples of such a goddess is the goddess Hāritī who is linked to Buddhist and Hindu traditions. She is said to have killed and eaten children but later becomes a protector of children. (Samuel 2008, 247–248). More prominent goddesses such as Śītalā (in North India) and Māriyammaṇ (in South India) are "fever goddesses," particularly linked to smallpox and other fever diseases requiring propitiation through rituals and sometimes through animal sacrifice to remove the contagion (Srinivas 2020; Yadav 2022). Plague Amma, or Black Māriyammaṇ, becomes the patron goddess of the plague in parts of South India (Muralidharan 2021; Srinivas 2020). More recently, we have seen the emergence of goddesses such as "Aids Amma" (Birkenholtz 2018; Srinivas 2020) as well as figures such as "Traffic Circle Amma" (Srinivas 2020).

6 Kāmātcipuṟam Ādhīnam and Plague Māriyammaṉ Temples in Coimbatore

In June 2020, a priest in Kerala built a shrine near his home and installed the first Corona Devi *mūrti* (icon) to ward off COVID-19 (Press Trust of India, 2021, Roychowdhury 2020). In May 2021, a Corona Devi *mūrti* was installed by Kāmātcipuṟam Ādhīnam Maṭh in the village of Irugur outside Coimbatore, Tamil Nadu. The installation of Corona Devi appeared in several media reports and across social media (Press Trust of India 2021). While the temple was not open to the public, the priests saw their actions as vital for the well-being of the community, with one temple trust member noting that deities like Corona Devi represent the "expression of the society and not that of the individual" (Press Trust of India, 2021). Several people tweeted short videos showing the consecration of the Corona Devi *mūrti* (deity statue) and snippets of the rituals available to the media. This temple is the latest addition to a complex of sixteen disease goddess temples in Coimbatore. Each of these is dedicated to Plague Māriyammaṉ (Black Māriyammaṉ),[11] who was thought to protect worshippers from earlier pandemics such as the plague and smallpox (Muralidharan 2021).

During 1903–1942, Coimbatore was affected by ten plague outbreaks, leading to the establishment of the Black Māriyammaṉ temples. They remained a source of solace during the subsequent smallpox and polio epidemics which racked India in the 1940s and 1950s. One of the women in the village, Kanammal, describes Black Māriyammaṉ's impact as follows:

> She is powerful, you know. It doesn't matter that we have a Corona Devi temple now. Black Māriammaṉ is one of us. We will continue to worship her, especially when we fall sick, but even for other kinds of general prayers too.
>
> (Muralidharan 2021)

Many in the region continue to believe that only Black Māriyammaṉ can stave off disease and put little stock in contemporary medicine, which was seen as ineffective in the face of these devastating diseases. Several residents believe that *pūjā* to the goddess would cure disease (Muralidharan 2021). One man who is a fourth-generation caretaker of a Black Māriyammaṉ temple in the region points to the longevity of the temples and the fact that no plague has impacted the region since the temple's consecration as a marker of its efficacy. He notes:

> This temple has been in existence for over 150 years. When the plague visited Coimbatore [1903–1942], my great-grandfather decided to consecrate an additional idol as Plague Mariamman. After him, my

> grandfather and my father took care of it. I do it today. Since then, no region under the reign of the goddess has been affected by plague. And so people have continued to have faith in her.
>
> (Muralidharan 2021)

7 The Viral Twitter Campaign for Pandemic Deities

In May 2020, in the Nichupara Basti of Asansol, West Bengal, women offered *pūjā* to "Corona Mai/Maa," another name for "Corona Devi." Similar rituals sprang up in Uttar Pradesh, Assam, Tamil Nadu, and Kerala in May–August 2020 and continued through the following year (Samanta 2020). There were three main ways in which Corona Devi manifests: (1) rural communities of women in Uttar Pradesh, Bihar, Assam, West Bengal, Kerala, and Tamil Nadu offered mantras and *pūjā* to Corona Devi; (2) *Paṇḍāls* in West Bengal during Durga *pūjā* transformed Durgā into a destroyer of Coronasur; (3) a temple was erected to Corona Devi in Tamil Nadu; a priest installed a shrine to Corona Devi in Kerala. In an age of "instant media," nothing could remain confined within national borders, much like the pandemic itself (Ramaswamy and Kaur 2020, 88). In this sense, it seems inevitable that the images and rituals of Corona Devi/Corona Mai would become a part of the digital media ecosphere.

My analysis focuses on tweets of media reports of Corona Devi rituals in villages located in West Bengal, Uttar Pradesh, Kerala, Bihar, the temple erected in Coimbatore, and the burning of the effigy of Coronasur in Mumbai. These reports are based on interviews with women in villages and small cities who perform rituals to Corona Mai/Corona Devi to stave off the virus, temple priests, or observations by journalists. Approximately a year after the initial reports of rituals to Corona Devi, we see media reports and tweets detailing the emergence of a Corona Devi temple in Coimbatore, Tamil Nadu.

8 Representative Tweets

Here are some representative English-language tweets on the opening of Corona Devi temples and Corona Devi rituals being performed in various parts of India. These tweets are a sampling of thousands of tweets that show images, videos, or feature descriptions of rituals to Corona Devi/Corona Mai. The term "Coronasur" only appears sparsely in reference to media stories about the burning of the Coronasur effigy in Mumbai.

1. "This #TamilNadu #temple got a **#CoronaDevi** idol to protect people from Covid. In the wake of the coronavirus crisis, Kamatchipuri Adhinam has decided to use granite to create the Corona Devi #deity and

conduct special prayers for 48 days"[12] (@sandipseth). This tweet shows a video of a temple consecration ceremony for Corona Devi.

2 "Now Indians believing in #CoronaDevi.... Hinduism already have 86000 Devi and Devtas, why not one more. I personally feel they should elect #CoronaDevi as Pm of India. She might do more Good than @ narendramodi. And at least won't commit The Holocaust in Indian Occupied Kashmir" (@essell1).[13] This tweet shows the Kāmātchipuṟam Ādhīnam temple consecration ceremony for Corona Devi. It has 83 likes, 19 retweets, and 5 comments.

3 "After #BodyguardMuneeswarar & #PlagueMariamman, it's #CoronaDevi's time in TN 😌😌 Coimbatore Kamatchipuri Aadhinam established Corona Devi Temple for the well-being of the people. #JaiCoronaDevi" (@suchisoundlover).[14] This tweet shows a video of the temple installation of Corona Devi, 85 views.

4 "After #blackmariamman, now Coimbatore is famous for Corona Devi temple. Kamatchipuri Adhinam has created and consecrated 'Corona Devi,' a deity dedicated to protecting people from #COVID19 #CoronaDevi #Coimbatore @News18TamilNadu" (@mahajournalist).[15] This tweet from a verified Twitter account shows a video of the temple ceremony for Corona Devi, which was viewed 9,649 times, has 70 likes, and 24 quote retweets.

5 "Shameful! It happens only in India #Covid_19 #CoronaDevi" (@ kartickrastogi). This tweet includes an image with text which reads: 'Coronavirus Pandemic | Solapur's Pardhi community refuses to wear masks, claims Corona Devi will protect them. For the past few months, the Pardhi community in Barshi town have been sacrificing chicken and goats and offering them to the new-found goddess Corona Devi, seeking her blessings to protect them from COVID-19,' September 3, 2020 by Moneycontrol News.[16] This tweet represents several similar critiques of Corona Devi veneration, which express concern that non-medical solutions to the pandemic would proliferate.

6 "I'm a native of Coimbatore, Tamilnadu. I am proud of my place for 1000 reasons, but this is not one of them. Corona Devi temple? Seriously? Nothing wrong in this per se, but I hope that people don't throng the temple with a hope that Covid will go away 🙏 #CoronaDevi #Coimbatore," Quote Tweet: @ANI, May 20, 2021: "Tamil Nadu: Priests offer special prayer to 'Corona Devi' in a temple in Coimbatore to contain the spread of #COVID19 'We are continuously praying to 'Corona Devi' to show mercy on us and help us get rid of this virus,' said Temple Priest" (@PraveenIFShere).[17] This tweet, which expresses concern that temple installations will prompt "temple throngs" and another wave of infections, includes a link to ANI news coverage of the Corona Devi temple in Coimbatore. It was liked 54 times and retweeted four times.

7 "(New Goddess introduced in INDIA) From West Bengal, #India, people found a new way to defeat #coronavirus. They started to pray a

new goddess they call "#CoronaDevi" or "#CoronaMai," which should protect people who praise her from #Covid_19 infection" (@BilalAkbar07).[18] This tweet shows an image of women in a West Bengal village performing a ritual to Corona Devi/Corona Mai.

8 "One more to the list of India's 330 million Gods & Goddesses. A New Temple for the New Goddess: 'Corona Devi'" (@ashoswai).[19] This tweet, from a verified account, shows an image from the consecration ceremony of Corona Devi in the Kāmātchipuṟam Adhinam temple complex in Coimbatore. The tweet has 1,515 likes, 74 quote retweets, and 356 retweets.

9 "Amid the global #pandemic in #Bihar, '#CoronaDevi' has emerged as a goddess for village women who believe it would rid them of the corona infection" (@NH_India).[20] This tweet, from a verified news organization, covers the worship of Corona Devi/Corona Mai/Corona Mātā in Bihar.

10 "#Superstitions galore: Now, '#CoronaDevi' emerges in #Bihar http://owl.li/IRKN30qNdkG" (@yespunjab).[21] This tweet shows an image of women conducting a Corona Devi/Corona Mai ritual in Bihar.

11 "#कोरोना (#Corona) #देवी की जय (Victory to the #Goddess) #कोरोनादेवी (#Coronadevi) #CoronaDevi #pujas held to ward off #coronavirus, #superstition sends Twitter into a frenzy http://dhunt.in/9UIa6?s=a&uu=0x3c2010bfcde664de&ss=pd Source: 'India TV' via Dailyhunt Download Now http://dhunt.in/DWND" (@urjaking).[22] While I focused on my tweet search on English-language hashtags and terms (e.g., "Corona Devi" and "Corona Mai"), the multilingual hashtags in this tweet show the reciprocal relationship between analog rituals and Twitter networks by linking to a news story which cites tweets in Hindi and English and shows videos of Corona Devi rituals taking place in rural regions of Bihar, parts of Jharkhand, West Bengal, and Uttar Pradesh.

12 "people, mostly women, r now performing '#CoronaDevi Puja' in #Assam #india. Dey believe that it is the only way to put an end of the deadly coronavirus pandemic: https://www.indiatoday.in/amp/india/story/assam-corona-Devi-pūjā-coronavirus-1686334-2020-06-06" (@gulaboo39).[23] This tweet links to an *India Today* story (verified media outlet), also shared by several other Twitter users, on women in rural Assam who perform rituals to Corona Devi and claim no one in their village succumbed to the virus as a result.

9 Tweet Analysis and Findings

Here are a few observations regarding the tweets I have chosen to include: (1) I focused on representative tweets with the hashtags and search terms #CoronaDevi and #CoronaMai and the volume of these tweets; (2) Most of these posts have only a few likes and shares, with the most engagement being 1,515 likes and 430 retweets/quote retweets. (3) These tweets were selected according to a topic, chronology, and term usage. (4) I chose tweets representing similar or identical tweets that were posted, which suggests that media reports that covered the rituals to Corona Devi in rural villages in West Bengal, Uttar Pradesh, Bihar, and Assam in 2020 and the temple installation of Corona Devi in Coimbatore in 2021 were being reproduced widely online.

Nearly every tweet that discussed the consecration of Corona Devi in the temple complex run by Kāmātcipuṟam Ādhīnam Maṭh displays an image or video of the ceremony taken from a media report. This suggests that the overall corpus of posts which share media reports rather than the liking or retweeting posts is most important for the proliferation of Corona Devi/Corona Mai going viral. In other words, many users were posting about this, but they were not necessarily in the same Twitter networks. This phenomenon spotlights an important nuance in how virality works on social media. Some viral campaigns are manufactured by a single user or group of users who can coordinate the use of a hashtag through verified accounts (see most politician and celebrity accounts). In the case of the Corona Devi/Corona Mai virtual corpus, these posts mostly come from individual users without large followings who are interacting with news reports about a phenomenon rather than each other. Most tweets, comments, and quote tweets show the importance of the analog ritual. In a few cases (see examples 1, 6, 8, and 10), they ridicule the use of rituals as superstition or critique government policies of virus mitigation seen as an impetus for such rituals. One tweet (6) expresses concern that the consecration of Corona Devi in a temple will lead to "throngs" within the temple. Even such a concern recognizes the importance physical places of worship hold for most Hindus.

My analysis shows that during the pandemic, despite the fact that temples did hold audio chanting, Facebook live *pūjā*, and other online access to sacred rites, prayers performed in physical temples remained authoritative for Hindu adherents. Moreover, the push to reopen temples dovetails with concerns about financial hardship, despite fears regarding subsequent waves of infection. This tracks with a Pew Research study's findings, which show that belief in God does not wane in the face of financial hardship:

> Indians who have had financial difficulties in the previous year (i.e., had trouble paying for food, medical care or housing) are similar to other Indians in how they interact with and believe in God – even when the actions or beliefs touch on financial matters. For example, Indians who have faced financial hardship are about as likely to ever ask God for prosperity (94%) as they are to ask for good health (93%) or forgiveness (92%).
>
> (Sahgal et al. 2021)

Virtual networks have provided opportunities for religious expression, the building of community, and even spiritual engagement since the early 2000s. Social media platforms have both enhanced the reach of traditional brick-and-mortar religious institutions (Åhman and Thorén 2021) as well as created new types of integration between online and offline spaces (Campbell and Lövheim 2011; Zeiler 2020). Spaces like Twitter can provide the kind of "connectivity" Van Dijck points out is central to the ethos of the platform in decentralized ways that impact offline activities and behaviors (Van Dijck 2013). Specifically, individuals and organizations that are not influencers on Twitter still can have a collective impact on offline communities of practice even when their posts are not connecting to a broader community or with each other. In the case of Corona Devi/Corona Mai, two themes emerge: 1) Corona Devi rituals in physical sacred spaces remain important as part of fighting COVID-19; 2) Economy and health are connected for Hindu adherents through the worship of Corona Devi. Thus, fighting the virus means a return to both physical and economic well-being.

In this sense, we see the online tweet corpus directing users to the physical space. This dovetails with the concerns of religious authorities in India, who saw physical places of worship as vital (Press Trust of India 2020). As one priest wrote in a letter to Prime Minister Narendra Modi in a bid to reopen temples, "If all temples, shrines and pilgrimage centres are reopened, the coronavirus cannot do any harm" (Press Trust of India 2020). Such an argument has both religious and economic implications. The lockdown in India lasted two months (March–May 2020) before businesses, schools, places of worship, and other public enterprises were allowed to reopen. Lockdown measures severely hampered the Indian economy, exacerbating poverty and straining social welfare programs that were already struggling to provide support (Gupta et al. 2021). Indeed, as Ravinder Kaur and Sumathi Ramaswamy note, "the biological threat posed by the virus was merged with the political-economic threat posed by the world's second-largest economy to the national well-being" (Ramaswamy and Kaur 2020). In this sense, Corona Devi offers a salve for these twinned impacts of COVID-19, a spiritual solution with an economic benefit.

Temples are part of a robust religion industry in India that was valued at $40 billion dollars in 2020, with half of that attributed to Hindu places of worship and spiritual/ritual practices and with the bulk of that wealth coming from informal labor markets (Nagaraj 2020; Sundaram 2021). In this sense, the case to reopen temples has purchase within both religious and economic spheres. As one priest noted, "the closure of temples has also adversely impacted the economic condition of priests" (Press Trust of India 2020). However, the economic condition of priests is far better than those who rely on the temple such as daily wage laborers, purveyors of ritual items, and sanitation workers who were unable to work during the lockdown. Indeed, one shopkeeper whose family sold Hindu ritual items for generations could not imagine closing his store on the eve of a festival. "For the first time, there will be no rush at my store before Gudi Padwa, and I am so shocked that I have not been able to even comprehend how it will impact my business in the coming months" (Nagaraj 2020).

10 Conclusion: How Corona Devi's Digital Fame Justifies the Need for Analog Sacred Spaces

Although the pandemic did inspire digital innovations that unsettle the notion of the analog sacred space as the center of authoritative ritual practice, the emergence of Corona Devi, one of the most prominent and visible religious icons during the COVID-19 pandemic, reinforces the importance of the physical temple for both lay practitioners and religious leaders. Even when religious leaders questioned the wisdom of opening temples with rising COVID-19 cases, the virtual queues for temples immediately filled (Varma et al. 2020). Hindu ritual websites, which proliferated before and during the pandemic, require analog temples for their business models. These websites are essentially broker sites in which a devotee can purchase a ritual, which is then performed (in most cases) in a physical temple. Many ritual websites experienced delays and even suspended services in some cases during the lockdown as access to physical temples was limited (Sundaram 2021). However, the analog rituals for Corona Devi emerge within these physical realities of the pandemic. The figure of Corona Devi acts as a bulwark against COVID-19 only when those the virus impacts perform the rituals in the place where it is rampant. These rituals are performed by women in rural communities who remain distrustful of government-run healthcare facilities which had developed an ominous reputation of admitting the sick and returning only their bodies. The later installation of the Corona Devi image as part of the Kāmātcipuṟam Ādhīnam Maṭh and temple complex in Coimbatore represents the vitality and efficacy that Hindu adherents continue to attach to physical sacred spaces, even when the devotees themselves cannot attend rituals.

Moreover, the Twittersphere, which documents the rituals of both temple priests and rural worshippers of Corona Devi, amplifies their practices and thereby reaffirms their authority but does not alter them fundamentally. In this sense, Stewart Hoover's point about authority as "something that is also constructed" is useful (Hoover 2016, 32). It is true that physical sacred spaces have held sway in Hindu traditions. However, in the case of Corona Devi, the deity's authority was, as Hoover argues, a "received authority [that] has a necessary precedence in the making of religious meanings...[and] can have some claim through its authenticity—or assumed authenticity—in the cultural marketplace" (Hoover 2016, 32). He also notes that "authority does rest to an extent in the individuals and groups who are active in imbricating these various sources, as well as in new networks of shared value that emerge from media (and particularly digital) practice" (Hoover 2016, 32). In other words, the virtual public of Twitter becomes a place in which religious authority is tested, negotiated, and, in this case, reaffirmed as indelibly linked to the analog world. As the worship of Corona Devi goes "viral," every post emphasizes the belief that analog rituals for and offerings to Corona Devi in the form of the wind or the sun or later as a *mūrti* remain paramount. In this sense, Twitter's virtual networks reinforce the authority of physical sacred space rather than undermining or relocating it. The tweets draw attention to how these communities are coping with a calamity for which healthcare professionals, politicians, and religious leaders were unable to solve. The women who perform these rituals are poor, have little access to private healthcare, and are often in remote or underserved regions of India. As the cited tweets show, these women were media subjects, not agents—they were not creating threads on Twitter or sharing their rituals online. The temple priests, though holding both caste and class privilege, also were not tweeting about the installation of Corona Devi in a temple. However, as observers and media outlets make these rituals go viral, the dual impact of temple closures on economic and physical wellness becomes clear. The rituals to Corona Devi offer the only solution accessible to communities that did not have the luxury of avoiding the virus and an effective measure in combatting it even for those who could worship virtually.

Notes

1 Nabil Echchaibi and Stewart Hoover describe "third spaces" in digital religion "as important performative sites of enunciation where formal and unitary structures of religious knowledge and practice become the object of both revision and transformation" (Hoover and Echchaibi 2014, 17). I use this idea to consider how the Twitter discourse of Corona Devi/Corona Mai leverages the in-betweenness of social media such that the digital practice of materiality transforms and in this case, provides ground for the the importance of physical, offline sacred spaces.

2 I do not use diacritics for "Corona Devi" since the term is used commonly without them.

3 Throughout this piece, I will use the terms "physical," "analog," and "offline" interchangeably to discuss religious spaces and activities in opposition to "digital," "virtual," or "online" spaces to highlight the divide between sacred activities in digital modalities versus those in analog spaces.

4 The term *asur* refers to a malevolent being with divine powers in Brahmanical Hinduism which is sometimes translated as "demon."

5 Most of the tweets I examined are in English though many tweets in Hindu, Bengali, Tamil, and Malayalam also display the hashtags #CoronaDevi and #CoronaMai. I do not cite these tweets, but they are part of the overall corpus and show the broad reach of these hashtags within the social media ecosphere.

6 Māriyammaṉ (goddess of smallpox) is the South Indian counterpart to the North Indian deity Śītalā (fever goddess). Māriyammaṉ is also worshipped by agricultural communities to bring rain to help crops flourish.

7 While it is not possible to know the identity and location of posters with certainty, the perspective and positionality the tweets espouse indicate an outsider perspective. For example, none of the tweets have language that suggest that the poster was conducting the ritual, participating in the ritual, or witnessing the ritual live.

8 *Dīkṣatar*-s are Brahman priests that train and help place priests within temples across a region. They are seen as authorities on theological issues and interpretations of canonical, orthodox, Brahmanical Hindu traditions.

9 The term *karmabhūmi* refers to the land space of India which is considered powerful and divine. Rituals and worship conducted within this physical space have authority and efficacy according to orthodox Hindu traditions.

10 These data on application access are taken from the application webpages and viewership information is available through Google analytics.
11 In Tamil "māri" also means "black" which is why this this name is used to describe Māriyamman.
12 Sandeep Seth, Tweet, May 19, 2021, https://twitter.com/sandipseth/status/1395011774181625860.
13 Dewan Sachal, Tweet, May 27, 2021, https://twitter.com/essel1/status/1397863491537616896.
14 Suchithra Seetharaman, Tweet, May 19 2021, https://twitter.com/suchisoundlover/status/1395008854480457735.
15 Mahalingam Ponnusamy, Tweet, May 19, 2021, https://twitter.com/mahajournalist/status/1394972447842111494
16 Kartick Rastogi, Tweet, September 3, 2020, https://twitter.com/KARTICKRASTOGI/status/1301526287056400386.
17 Praveen Angusamy, IFS, Tweet, May 21, 2021, https://twitter.com/PraveenIFShere/status/1395591923427987456
18 Bilal Akbar, July 12, 2020, https://twitter.com/BilalAkbar07/status/1282329585808543745.
19 Ashok Swain, May 22, 2021, https://twitter.com/ashoswai/status/1396003733276971011.
20 National Herald, Tweet, June 6, 2020, https://twitter.com/NH_India/status/1269254448615915520.
21 YesPunjab.com, Tweet, June 6, 2020, https://twitter.com/yespunjab/status/1269223424892821506.
22 Yogesh Divekar, Tweet, June 7, 2020, https://twitter.com/urjaking/status/1269566694789275650.
23 Ghazala, Tweet, June 8, 2020, https://twitter.com/gulaboo39/status/1269776708523167745.

Bibliography

Åhman, Henrik and Claes Thorén, "When Facebook Becomes Faithbook: Exploring Religious Communication in a Social Media Context," *Social Media + Society*, (7) 3 (2021): 1–12.

Birkenholtz, Jessica V. *Reciting the Goddess*, London, New York: Oxford University Press, 2018.

Campbell, Heidi and Mia Lövheim, "Rethinking the Online–Offline Connection in the Study of Religion Online," *Information, Communication & Society*, (14) 8 (2011): 1083–1096.

Cheong, Pauline, "Tweet the Message? Religious Authority and Social Media Innovation," *Journal of Religion, Media and Digital Culture*, (3) 3 (2014): 1–19.

Chowdhury, Srimoyee. "Durga Idol Reimagined as Doctor Killing 'Coronasur' Goes Viral, Shashi Tharoor Praises It," *Hindustan Times*, Accessed on February 22, 2022, October 20, 2020, https://www.hindustantimes.com/it-s-viral/durga-idol-reimagined-as-doctor-killing-coronasur-goes-viral-shashi-tharoor-praises-it/story-hIfspIck9HHKlrjF6rrbHO.html.

Dudrah, Rajinder, Sangita Gopal, Amit Rai, and Anustup Basu (eds.), *InterMedia in South Asia The Fourth Screen*, London: Routledge, 2012.

Eck, Diana, *Banaras: City of Light*, New York: Alfred A. Knopf, 1982.

Evolvi, Guilia, "Materiality, Authority, and Digital Religion: The Case of a Neo-Pagan Forum," *Entangled Religions* (11) 3 (2020), 1–15.

Granoff, Phyllis and Koichi Minohara, *Pilgrims, Patrons, and Place: Localizing Sanctity in Asian Religions*, Vancouver: University of British Columbia Press, 2007.

Gupta, Vendika, K. C. Santosh, Rameshwar Arora, Tiziana Ciano, Khairul S. Kalid, and Senthilkumar Mohan, "Socioeconomic Impact Due to COVID-19: An Empirical Assessment," *Information Process and Management Journal* (online) (59) 2 (2021), https://www.sciencedirect.com/science/article/pii/S0306457321002855.

Hoover, Stewart M. and Nabil Echchaibi, Media Theory and "the 'Third Spaces' of Digital Religion," in *Finding Religion in the Media: Work in Progress on the Third Spaces of Digital Religion*, edited by Stewart Hoover and Nabil Echchaibi, Boulder: Center for Media, Religion, and Culture, 2014, 1–35.

Hoover, Stewart M., "Religious Authority in the Media Age," in *The Media and Religious Authority*, edited by Stewart Hoover, University Park: Penn State University Press, 2016, 15–36.

Hudson, Dennis, *The Body of God: An Emperor's Palace for Krishna in Eighth-Century Kanchipuram*, New York: Oxford University Press, 2008.

Hutchings, Tim and Joanne McKenzie, *Materiality and the Study of Religion: The Stuff of the Sacred*, New York: Routledge, 2016.

Lang, Natalie, "Saint Corona, CoronAsur, and Corona Devi: New Embodiments of the Relationship between Religion and Disease," (blog) *CoronAsur Research Blog*, Asia Research Institute, Accessed on April 3, 2022, July 3, 2020, https://ari.nus.edu.sg/20331-25/.

Mahadeva Diksatar, interview by Dheepa Sundaram, Bangalore, Karnataka, December 12, 2018.

Meyer, Birgit, "Religious Sensations: Why Media, Aesthetics and Power Matter in the Study of Contemporary Religion," in *Religion Beyond a Concept*, edited by Hent de Vries, New York: Fordham University Press, 2008, 704–723.

Mitra, Piyali, "Religion and COVID-19," (blog) Woolf Institute, Accessed on June 2, 2022, May 12, 2020, https://www.woolf.cam.ac.uk/blog/religion-and-covid-19-in-india.

Muralidharan, Kavita, "In Coimbatore: Death, Disease and Divinity," (blog) *People's Rural Archive of India*, Accessed on May 20, 2022, November 11, 2021, https://ruralindiaonline.org/or/articles/in-coimbatore-death-disease-and-divinity/.

Nagaraj, Anuradha, "From Flowers to Incense, India's Temple Economy Hit by Coronavirus," *Reuters*, Accessed on June 1, 2022, March 24, 2020, https://www.reuters.com/article/us-health-coronavirus-festival-india/from-flowers-to-incense-indias-temple-economy-hit-by-coronavirus-idUSKBN21C075.

Press Trust of India, "Coimbatore Now Has a Temple for 'Corona Devi'," *The Economic Times*, Accessed on March 23, 2022, May 21, 2021, https://economictimes.indiatimes.com/news/india/coimbatore-now-has-a-temple-for-corona-devi/corona-devi-temple/slideshow/82855588.cms.

Press Trust of India, "Corona an 'Asur' Can Only Be Killed by Divine Forces, Says Priests Body; Seeks Temple Reopening," *Business-Standard*, Accessed on February 1, 2022, May 12, 2020, https://www.business-standard.com/article/pti-stories/corona-an-asur-can-only-be-killed-by-divine-forces-says-priests-body-seeks-temple-reopening-120051600777_1.html.

Ramaswamy, Sumathi and Ravinder Kaur, "The Goddess and the Virus," in *Pandemic: Perspectives on Asia*, edited by Vinayak Chaturvedi, New York: Columbia University Press, 2020, 75–94.

Roychowdhury, Adrija, "When Fear Leads to Faith: The Disease Gods of India," *Indian Express*, Accessed on June 2, 2022, June 22, 2020, https://indianexpress.com/article/research/when-fear-leads-to-faith-the-disease-gods-of-india-6470376/.

Sahgal, Neha, Jonathan Evans, Ariana Monique Salazar, Kelsey Jo Starr, and Manolo Corichi, "Religious Practices," Pew Research Center, Accessed on April 10, 2022, June 29, 2021, https://www.pewresearch.org/religion/2021/06/29/religious-practices-2/.

Samanta, Sanchari, "How a Goddess Called Corona Devi Came To Be Worshipped in West Bengal," *The Hindu*, Accessed on June 1, 2022, June 10, 2020, https://www.thehindu.com/society/a-goddess-called-corona-devi/article31795320.ece.

Samuel, Geoffrey, *The Origins of Yoga and Tantra; Indic Religions to the Thirteenth Century*, Cambridge: Cambridge University Press, 2008.

Slater, Joanna and Niha Masih, "In India's Surge, a Religious Gathering Attended by Millions Helped the Virus Spread," *The Washington Post*, Accessed on February 24, 2022, May 8, 2021, https://www.washingtonpost.com/world/2021/05/08/india-coronavirus-kumbh-mela/.

Srinivas, Tulasi, "India's Goddesses of Contagion Provide Protection in the Pandemic – Just Don't Make Them Angry," (blog) *Pandemic Response and Religion in the USA: Doctrine* (34), Accessed on November 14, 2020, June 15, 2020, https://scholarworks.wmich.edu/religion-pandemic-doctrine/34.

Sundaram, Dheepa, "Digitizing Sacred Spaces: How COVID-19 Fueled Innovation of Hindu Ritual Websites," *Religion News Service*, Accessed on October 28, 2021, October 28, 2021, https://religionnews.com/2021/10/28/digitizing-sacred-spaces-how-covid-19-has-fueled-innovation-of-hindu-ritual-websites/.

Van Dijck, José, *Cultural of Connectivity: A Critical Historiography of Social Media*, London: Oxford University Press, 2013.

Varma, Vishnu, Ralph Alex Arakal, BP Darshan Devaiah, Tora Agarwala, and Sonakshi Awasthi, "As Places of Worship Reopen Across India, the Moot Question Remains: Is It Safe?," *Indian Express*, Accessed on February 22, 2022, June 8, 2020, https://indianexpress.com/article/india/unlock-1-places-of-worship-temples-mosques-open-6449151/.

Yadav, Megha, "Disease, Demon, and the Deity: Case of Corona Mātā and Coronāasur in India," *Religions* (13) 1011 (2022), 1–13.

Young, Glenn, "Reading and Praying Online: The Continuity of Religion Online and Online Religion in Internet Christianity," in *Religion Online: Finding Faith on the Internet*, edited by L. Dawson and D.E. Cowan, London: Routledge, 2004, 93–106.

Zeiler, Xenia, "Introduction," in *Digital Hinduism*, edited by Xenia Zeiler, London: Routledge, 2020, 1–10.

3 Sitting on a Grave

Female Agency and Resistance during the COVID-19 Pandemic in Chiga Village, Kenya

Loreen Maseno

1 Introduction

COVID-19 in Kenya necessitated an enforcement of Ministry of Health (MOH) burial guidelines. These were met with resistance at various levels, even as the State demanded that these guidelines be unilaterally enforced. After the community of Chiga village was outwitted by the security agents, it took two women's agency to save the day. The severe acute respiratory syndrome (SARS) COVID-19 was identified as causing a cluster of pneumonia and deaths in Wuhan city, China on December 31, 2019. In recent times, it has continued to cause morbidity and mortalities due to its rapid spread to other parts of the world, Kenya not being exempted. The World Health Organization (WHO) declared COVID-19 a pandemic. Between 83,000 and 190,000 people in Africa could die of COVID-19 and 29 million to 44 million could get infected during the pandemic if containment measures fail.[1] The predicted number of cases that would require hospitalization would overwhelm the available medical capacity in much of Africa. There would be an estimated 3.6 million–5.5 million COVID-19 hospitalizations, of which 82,000–167,000 would be severe cases requiring oxygen and 52,000–107,000 would be critical cases requiring breathing support.[2] COVID-19 as a pandemic has greatly impacted communities worldwide. The measures put in place include social distancing and the discouraging of gatherings embedded within the customs of the people of Kenya and which have of old been useful.

COVID-19 continues to be presented as an existential threat, justifying alternative actions outside the usually prescribed procedure. This essay adopts securitization theory to critically examine the existential threat and measures through which the MOH prescribes the conduct of burial ceremonies in Kenya. Additionally, physical access to health services is very restricted to the general population, so that many people would not even have the chance to access medical care if they needed it. In spite of these glaring challenges, female agency has a role to play during this pandemic and demonstrable in various forms. This paper locates the agency around burials and, by using one case in the public domain of Kenya, argues that two

DOI: 10.4324/b22930-4

women sitting on a grave were able to accomplish what state security agencies could not enforce and maintain. This essay is a feminist reflection on an event in which the mother and wife of Jachiga sat on the grave in defiance of a call by predominantly male villagers to exhume the dead after a hurried and securitized state-managed burial done in the night. Sitting on the grave is a localized and dramatic her-story that showcases resilience and captures the state's inadequacies in addressing current COVID-19 burial-related stalemates and lessons. This essay uses the concepts of female agency, power, and securitization to present and analyze these happenings during the COVID-19 pandemic in Kenya.[3] This chapter will provide a background of the COVID-19 pandemic in Kenya and further highlight the context of Luo funeral rites and burial traditions in Kenya. It shall bring to sharp focus Jachiga's death and funeral within the terrain of securitization of COVID-19 and funerals. The resistance of the two women serves to exemplify the female agency

2 The COVID-19 Pandemic in Kenya

Upon the arrival of COVID-19 in Kenya, the first death cases were reported in March 2019. There has been a total of 1,072 deaths as of November 2020 out of 59,595 confirmed cases of COVID-19.[4] Many deaths have evoked fear and uncertainty about the proper disposal of human remains. At the start of the pandemic, any patient with breathing complications who then passed away was to be buried within 24 hours. Burial ceremonies were securitized to ensure that as few people as possible were in attendance and that no food was served to people at the gathering. At the same time, securitization ensured that, under the gaze of the police and other security apparatus, the MOH guidelines were adhered to and that no corpse would be touched or viewed by mourners.

3 Luo Funeral Rites and Burial Traditions

The southern Luo who practice Luo culture are of Nilotic origin. Dholuo is the language spoken by groups of people in Sudan, Ethiopia, Congo, Uganda, Kenya, and Tanzania.[5] The Luo are patrilineal; senior members stand in the highest position in the kinship value hierarchy.[6] Besides external influences, there have been internal transformations within Luo culture itself, for example, from a fishing and nomadic society to a settled mixed agricultural one. Luo culture provides the Luo people with the symbols, language, beliefs, and attitudes to make sense of their world.[7]

Luo culture and society extend over diverse territories. Yet, this multiplicity informs Luo people with norms to live by and how to structure social relations. Questions regarding people's well-being and their status are explained within the ever-changing framework of culture. According to the Luo custom of marriage, death alone does not dissolve a marriage contract. A widow still remains the legal wife of her deceased man and may be expected to have further children to his name through leviratic relationships. In that case, a close kinsman of the dead man, in the line of brother-in-law *Yuore*, may take on the role of caretaker.[8]

In all human cultures, death is considered a devastating moment and generally met with a lot of emotions. Death rituals among the Luo take center stage and bear deep effects on the widow and her children. Gunga suggests that, apart from the survivor's feelings of loss and the physical absence of the deceased person, death means no particular harm for the dead person per se because the idea is that one reverts to the prenatal state similar to before birth.[9] This position is questionable, however, when it is related to status and rank among the Luo, because ancestors, the living dead, the living, the unborn, etc. are all conceptualized as guardians of human morality. The unborn, therefore, cannot be equated with the dead.[10]

Bereavement among the Luo involves rituals and harassment; like in many other African cultures, it also places restrictions on the surviving partner. Ethnographic information from a neighboring community, the Abanyole, indicates that, upon the death of a spouse, a widow is being accompanied by a fellow widow to her native home and then expected to wail there so as to announce the death. Before the widow leaves to go to her parental home, the body of her late husband needs to have been removed from the house and put under a tent. While the body of her late husband is still under the tent, a widow cannot go to her parents' home. Upon her arrival at her parents' compound, the widow needs to wail loudly while entering the gate in order to alert the people in the homestead of the tragedy so that they do not greet her with gladness, as would be the custom.[11]

The death announcement is followed by the vigil (*budho*), for which relatives of the deceased stay awake within the compound for several nights until the actual burial day. According to Wakana Shiino, different songs from different Christian denominations, such as Catholic, Protestant, or New Religious movements like Roho, are also sung alongside lamentations depending on the religious affiliation of the family.[12] Luo rituals for the dead allow the living to express their sorrow while also providing an occasion for the display of the deceased person's prosperity, seniority, and greatness.[13]

According to Shiino, the Luo culture knows up to 14 rituals that need to be performed in successive order for each deceased person. Shiino further notes that there have been variations in recent times on how some rituals are done, in some cases because recent ancestors did not partake in the ritual or perhaps because of church teachings or even the eroding of cultural norms, so that people perform rituals the way they deem convenient to them.[14] With the state securitization of burials during the COVID-19 period, it is clear that all of these rituals could neither be done in their completeness nor in successive order. Due to these circumstances, problems arose when the musician popularly known as "Jachiga" deceased. His widow, Belinda, could not leave for her natal home since her husband's body had not yet been brought to their compound and placed under a tent. Nor could she wail, as this was a period of restrictions for gatherings. Due to that, a stalemate occurred between the security apparatus and the villagers, who are generally custodians of the traditions and cultural practices. It was unheard of that a deceased person should be brought from the mortuary and be buried on the same day; the Chiga villagers termed such a situation "burying a dog without respect." Villagers insisted, therefore, that they could not allow Jachiga to be buried within a day after his passing. He was their son and had to be given a decent burial. This they shouted as the locals refilled the grave, while others threw branches and iron sheets inside the dug grave.

According to the Luo, nothing happens without a cause, which is what their saying *Ok timre nono* conveys. Consequently, blame must be apportioned for either having broken *Kwer*,[15] or for having brought bad medicine into the village, or for having offended the ancestors. Therefore, the cause is determined as punishment either from God or from the spirits.[16] *Kwer* of higher levels implies offenses against the whole nation. Accordingly, the punishment is meted out to the whole society, such as defeat in war, famine, epidemics, and locusts. By contrast, *Kwer* of the lower level implies bringing *Chira*-sin consequences to individuals and their families, or perhaps their lineages.[17] It is within this cultural context that the stalemate between security agents and the mourners needs to be read. At the same time, the agency of the widow is heightened in this case. It magnifies her resistance following the death of her spouse.

According to Luo tradition, a widow takes part in *tero cholla*, a ritual that ends the mourning period. This is one of the spectrum of rituals that form part of sending off the dead in an honorable way. The widow was supposed to have in mind a man who would inherit her, and while she visited her natal home, this man was expected to sleep in her house for one night. Upon her return, the inheritor and the widow would eat meat that she had brought along from her natal home, and after that, they would have sex.[18]

4 Jachiga's Death

Benard Onyango was born in East Kolwa, Chiga Location, Kisumu County, in 1987. More popularly known as Jachiga Jachiga, he ventured into a musical career at the age of 21 as an instrumentalist. He was a husband and father of two. At the time of his demise, he was a popular Kisumu-based musician and bandleader who had only relocated to Nairobi less than two years prior. Jachiga was among the fast-rising popular musicians whose compositions were well received by fans both locally and in the diaspora. One of his popular Ohangla compositions was the '*Mano Kasinde*' chartbuster that took the local music industry by storm. Other songs he released include *Penzi Kama Yai*, *Nancy Nyarugenya,* and *Maraga Odagi.* The latter was influenced by the aftermath of the 2007 post-election violence in Kenya that saw hundreds of lives lost and property worth thousands of shillings destroyed.

According to K'olewe, Ohangla is modern Luo music, which is also part of the African traditional education, specifically oral literature (orature).[19]

To him, Ohangla should be seen in keeping with the goals of such education. As such, music plays an important role in the production of knowledge and the creation of a collective historical past. Through Ohangla, it is possible to problematize the orator and identity by raising questions about what it means to be part of the Luo community. According to Rose A. Omolo-Ongati, the Ohangla genre involves song and dance accompanied by an ensemble of four to eight tuned drums, distinguished by a long cylindrical drum (*ohangla*, or *kalapapla* in South Nyanza), from which it derives its name. These, together with the *ongeng'o* (a round metal ring struck with an iron rod), form the rhythmic base of the performance.[20]

Jachiga was mentored by the likes of Lady Maureen, another Luo music artist, and had a brief stay with Ohangla musician, Jakadenge, before he died. Jachiga went on to start his own band, which performed for several years at the former Gwara Gwara club in Kondele, Kisumu, Kenya. In mid-2018, after the release of his popular chartbusters, "*Mano Kasinde*" on an album with the same title, the musician and bandleader moved with his band to Nairobi in search of greener pastures. The song *Mano Kasinde* deals with the misuse of the word "cousin" and is borrowed from the English language to mean "her cousin." The song decries that unfaithful women in recent times have adopted the art of duping men by claiming every man they flirt with as their cousin.

Prior to his passing, it was reported that Jachiga silently suffered from pneumonia, which was on and off, although he always wore a brave face while in public. The report added that he had been frequenting the hospital during his battle with pneumonia for quite some time. According to medical doctors, the SARS virus affects the lungs and causes pneumonia-like symptoms in a patient. In these early days of the pandemic in the country, any chest infection, cough, etc. was publicly declared to be COVID-19 even prior to conclusive tests. Therefore, rumours spread that the virus could likely have been the cause of Jachiga's demise. During his final days, he was admitted to St. Elizabeth Hospital Kisumu before being transferred to St. Jairus Hospital. There, he lost the battle with his disease on Thursday, June 11, 2020, at 2:00 am. It is unfortunate that COVID-19 tests were carried out on Jachiga; however, the results returned sometime after the burial fiasco. It turned out that he was not COVID-19 positive. The assumption all along was that he died from COVID-19-related symptoms.[21]

5 Jachiga's Funeral

It was reported that one week after his death, fans came in large crowds to view the body of the musician, prompting the hospital administration to lock the gates, which later had to be secured by police. However, Jachiga disapproved of the measure and chased officers along the Kisumu-Busia Road in Kenya. The Kisumu Governor Anyang Nyong'o conveyed his condolences to the family of the musician, saying that Jachiga was an extremely talented musician who spent a lot of time mentoring young, upcoming musicians.

On the evening of Friday, June 13, 2020, hundreds of mourners defied police orders and public COVID-19 health guidelines as they escorted Jachiga's body for burial in the outskirts of Kisumu. Chanting funereal dirges, the mourners refused to maintain social distancing as ordered by police, and only a few wore face masks. In this way, the funeral procession moved from Kisumu's Port Florence Hospital mortuary to Chiga in Kisumu East subcounty.[22] A police convoy accompanied the hearse carrying Jachiga's body from the mortuary. On that occasion, thousands of mourners pelted police with stones, thus interrupting the burial. A police source said that the officers had been released from duty because they had suffered injuries. Efforts by police officers to restore order proved futile. The fans obtained the casket and kept it in their custody.

Mourners ensured that the casket was taken from the grave just before the police could cover it. The villagers insisted to walk with the casket around the village before taking it to near St. Elizabeth Chiga Missionary Hospital. According to some villagers, Jachiga had neither been accorded proper respect nor had his family or community been given enough time to grieve. Therefore, they would not stand aside and see him buried within 24 hours of his death. Villagers pelted the police convoys with stones and overpowered them; they also succeeded in refilling the grave and stopping any attempts to lay Jachiga to rest. One villager remarked: "They have dispersed us. They have tried to remove the soil from the grave and bury Jachiga, but we have refused. There will be no burial today." Exhausted and overwhelmed, the police officers retreated into the night.

It was reported that, after a long day of high drama and battles with the police, officers removed the body from the facility's morgue on Saturday at around 1:41 am. Only Jachiga's younger brother, Austin Omondi, whom the police called to identify the body at the morgue, was allowed to stand by the graveside at that time. A dusk to dawn curfew made it possible for the officers to carry out the burial at night. At 2:30 am, under tight security by police in plain clothes, Jachiga was hurriedly buried.

According to the musician's sister-in-law, Lillian Okello, the family was having a meeting during the night when they heard the sound of a police vehicle roaring toward the compound at about 1:51 am. "The casket was carried in one Land Cruiser with armed police officers. They ordered everyone to stay indoors despite many of us willing to pay our last respects to our loved one," said Mrs. Okello.

6 Securitization of COVID-19 and Funerals during COVID-19 in Kenya

Following the ravaging COVID-19 situation in Kenya, the MOH had to put up a raft of measures regarding the handling of bodies of deceased persons. Under the MOH guidelines, in Section 10 on the handling of human remains, burials in Kenya had to satisfy the following minimum requirements. First, burials had to be carried out strictly under the supervision of the Public Health Official (PHO)/Health Care Practitioner (HCP), and the disposal of remains of a human who had died from COVID-19 had to be overseen by a PHO. The process had to be concluded within 2 days (48 hours) to prevent community practices that would result in more infections through contact. Second, a health worker had to ensure that, during the handling of a casket, Personal Protective Equipment (PPE) is worn at all times. This guideline was to avoid the spread of the virus after the death of the patient. Third, upon sealing the corpse in a body bag, the latter was not be opened for viewing of the body thereafter. Fourth, the body had to be buried on the same day by the family under supervision of the HCP, the local health care committee leader, and religious leaders.

Fifth, relatives were strictly forbidden to touch or kiss the body, while the local health authorities had to designate a team to oversee the process of burials. These measures and more were set in motion at the onset of the pandemic in Kenya.

In the following, I will employ security theory to rethink this case. Developments in the field of securitization indicate that there are convergences between securitization and framing. Securitization is generally considered a subfield of framing in a movement toward 'security framing.'

7 Securitization Theory

Paul Bramadat considers securitization as the growing emphasis on national security, which may broadly be understood as increased international cooperation in the war on terror and narrowly as increased border controls for particular states.[23] Securitization has the effect of placing an agenda on the fore that is suggested to be of serious concern to the state or other actors. The theory of securitization explores the way a referent object (something) is deemed threatened and the security action necessary to defend or protect it. It examines the construction of threats and the implementation of policies thereafter. The Copenhagen School represents the body of work from Ole Weaver and Barry Buzan that focuses on linguistic-grammatical composition in the construction of security.[24]

Buzan understands securitization to include the process through which an issue such as COVID-19 is presented as an existential threat requiring urgent measures and justifies alternative actions outside the usually prescribed procedure.[25] Many alternative actions have been taken in Kenya after the reporting of the first COVID-19 case. Some of these actions include securitized burials, curfews across the country, disclosure of medical conditions, isolation, and quarantines. Furthermore, during funerals, health care personnel had been assigned to handle and lower caskets of persons they do not have any relation to. Securitization creates a second-order system useful in observing how main actors in the field of security studies operate. "It studies how security issues are produced by actors who pose something (a referent object) as existentially threatened and therefore claim a right to use an extraordinary measure to defend it."[26] The Cabinet Secretary to the ministry of health in Kenya had, on numerous occasions, warned that all Kenyans were existentially threatened unless they strictly adhered to the MOH protocols and guidelines. He has also instituted bylaws and laws that defended the measures issued, such as jail terms and sentences to persons who did not wear masks.

At the same time, securitization theory highlights the effects of securitization. Often times, referent objects are elevated to a level where their survival is threatened so much that if the threat is not dealt with swiftly, these objects will come to a point of no return or be destroyed.[27] Securitization theory, therefore, defines specifically four basic components:

First, securitizing actors who announce the security situation. They may range from cabinet secretaries and non-governmental organizations to activists, protectors, etc.[28] Since the pandemic has struck Kenya, there have been daily announcements from the MOH and the Cabinet secretaries on the number of persons who tested positive, how many have died, and how many have recovered. These announcements have been aired by leading television and radio outlets in Kenya. Furthermore, the print media have devoted large sections to COVID-19, the health systems' preparedness or unpreparedness, corruption in the sector, and deaths.

Second, the threat, which can be tangible like bombs, missiles, or intangible like a dangerous ideology. For the current study, the identified threat is COVID-19 and its rapid spread across the 47 counties of Kenya.[29] Third, the referent object, which is the target of the threat. This is the Kenyan populace who if not secured could lead to more deaths and the collapse of the entire Kenyan health system. Fourth, measures to actively deal with the impending threat.[30]

The process of securitization has also been deemed as a speech act in which the utterance itself is the act. It is by labeling something a security issue that it actually takes up the place to become one.[31] Moreover, the very act of referring to COVID-19 as a threat means securitizing it. The success in making the security move on matters of health for Kenyans and for which loss means death, ensured that priority was given to this pandemic than when attempting to securitize other objects.[32] Following the new rules by Kisumu Governor Anyang' Nyongó aimed at reducing the size of human crowds in the fight against the coronavirus, Jachiga's family was instructed to inter the body within 24 hours. In general, the mode of burial was no longer as detailed per African traditions and customs. This was rather distressing to the surviving family. The dead were not to be viewed anymore, even though it was the customary practice of ascertaining who is actually buried. The deceased family was barred from coming into direct contact with the dead. It has been argued, however, that this has the potential of destabilizing the deceased families' mental and spiritual health.[33] It turns out that burials could no longer be elaborate as African customs require. The government, as a securitizing actor, had highlighted the COVID-19 threat in relation to burials within the Kenyan context. It is clear that through securitization of COVID-19, human lives were deemed threatened and security actions were put in place to protect them.

8 Reading Female Agency and Resistance

Curfews had been imposed in Kenya since the advent of COVID-19 in March 2020. They have continued ever since, enforced by security agencies. On the Saturday morning after Jachiga's passing, villagers came to learn about the secret burial of Jachiga during the night. They became very agitated that it had been done without their participation.

Villagers stormed the home and demanded to exhume the body from the grave so as to bury Jachiga at a later date. However, his widow, Belinda Aluoch, and his mother, Monica Auma, decided to sit on the grave. They cried and demanded that they be killed first before they could allow the exhuming to begin. His mother shouted that the very act of exhuming him would kill her, and if this is what the villagers wanted, yet another death would occur in her home. The angry male villagers insisted that they were not sure whether the buried person was actually Jachiga since they had not participated in the funeral rites.

Both women refused to budge, saying that they would not get off the grave. Certain themes predominate in feminist discourse, one of which is the construction of personal agency. From a feminist perspective, the pervasive influence of this illusive dweller is related to the emphasis on individualism at the expense of context within traditional psychological models.[34] Belinda's sitting on the grave speaks volumes in the face of angry male villagers, whose ritual capital was eroded when they could not supervise and control the burial of one of theirs. Perhaps they saw themselves demeaned and rendered irrelevant in the deeply ritual process of burial in their village, hence their anger and disgust. They would have been sidelined in a way they were not comfortable with. The scene may indeed not have been about the widow and her deceased husband or her children, but about themselves.

Belinda and her mother-in-law managed to withstand the same villagers whom the police were unable to pacify with canisters and gunshots. The two declared that they would not budge. It was clear within the context that both demonstrated a capacity for individualized choice and action. According to Sharon Krause (2011), agency in feminist theory is proceeding along uncoupling the notions of agency and autonomy so as to propose a definition of agency as resilience in the face of coercion, oppression, and systematic marginalization.[35] To her, it is important to consider agency as a capacity for meaningful action rather than an unfettered individual choice. This interpretation takes into account structural inequality and injustice experienced by both Belinda and her mother-in-law but acknowledges that the women did not see this inequality or injustice as an insurmountable obstacle to agency.

Hence, agency is possible no matter how oppressed humans are or how attached to subordinating relations. At the same time, this case demonstrates the agency in others, regardless of personal privilege.

We take note that Belinda's resistance and agency are not equivalent to an autonomous choice in her context. According to Madhok et al., agency is to be seen as a mode of reflection. They add, "It is a way of taking responsibility for one's location in the world, a location that is not only or fully knowable by the subject." Belinda's actions are known by herself even as she sat on the grave along with her mother in law.[36]

9 Conclusion

COVID-19-related burial ceremonies in Kenya were securitized to ensure that they were conducted within the shortest time, under security personnel watch, and with the least number of people present. At the same time, securitization ensured that, under the gaze of police and other members of the security apparatus, the MOH guidelines of disposal of human remains were adhered to, and that the dead person was neither touched nor viewed by mourners. As a consequence, villagers and members of the public found their customs warped or disregarded. Furthermore, they were in fear of the spiritual implications of having an improper send-off for their loved ones. All of this was the case in the aggressive protest in Chiga Village, as discussed above. Though the government and MOH as actors have been in positions of political power, the Kenyan society found its own ways for agency and resistance.

Whereas news agencies focused on the battle between the state and the villagers, this essay shifted focus onto two women whose courage and agency ensured that the fallout between people's cultural burial rites and the state was settled. More of her-stories need to be brought to the limelight to show individual emancipation and freedom within the context of solidarity and belonging. It will be relevant to understand what empowers (and disempowers) individual women in contexts such as these. Sitting on the grave localizes a dramatic and potentially dangerous intervention by two women, a her-story that showcases the resilience and agency that left the late Jachiga resting.

Notes

1 WHO 2020; see https://covid19.who.int/
2 WHO 2020.
3 Cf. Collins, *Black Feminist Thought*; Collins, *Black Sexual Politics*; Gardiner, *Provoking Agents*; Laustsen and Wæver, "In Defence of Religion"; Buzan, Wæver, de Wilde, *Security*.
4 WHO 2020, online at https://covid19.who.int/region/afro/country/ke.
5 Cf. Ocholla-Ayayo, *Traditional Ideology*, 13.
6 Cf. Ocholla-Ayayo, *Traditional Ideology*, 39.
7 Cf. Odhiambo and Maseno, "Dramatic Irony."
8 Cf. Ocholla-Ayayo, *Traditional Ideology*, 144.

9 Cf. Gunga, "Politics," 167.
10 Cf. Ocholla-Ayayo, *Traditional Ideology*, 112.
11 Cf. Maseno-Ouma, *Abanyole African Widows*.
12 Cf. Shiino, "Death and Funeral Rituals," 215.
13 Ibid., 227.
14 Cf. Shiino, "Death and Funeral Rituals."
15 *Kwer* is equivalent to taboo.
16 Cf. Ocholla-Ayayo, *Traditional Ideology*, 113.
17 Cf. Ocholla-Ayayo, *Traditional Ideology*, 110.
18 Cf. Shiino, "Death and Funeral Rituals," 220.
19 K'Olewe, "*Benga* and *Ohangla* orature," 33–49.
20 Ongati, R. Recontextualization of *Orutu* Music of the Luo.
21 Once the tests results were released, in show of their sincere apology for handling the late Jachiga as one who had died from COVID-19, the top Officers Commanding Police Divisions came back to the home of the late with food supplies to give an apology to the family over what had transpired. This was in the full glare of the media. See https://www.standardmedia.co.ke/entertainment/the-standard/2001375847/police-visit-abenny-jachigas-family-bearing-gifts-apologize-over-burial-saga visited on 20.4.2022.
22 See https://www.standardmedia.co.ke/nyanza/article/2001374894/mourners-defy-police-covid-19-rules-to-escort-body-of-ohangla-musician.
23 Cf. Bramadat, "The Public, the Political and the Possible," 7–8.
24 Cf. Watson, Scott D., "'Framing' the Copenhagen School: Integrating Literature on Threat Construction," *Millennium: Journal of International Studies* 40, 2 (2012): 279–301.
25 Cf. Buzan, Wæver, de Wilde, *Security*, 24.
26 Laustsen and Wæver, "In Defence of Religion," 708.
27 Ibid.
28 Cf. Maseno, "Securitizing Places of Worship in Kenya."
29 Cf. Youde, "Who's Afraid of a Chicken?"
30 Cf. Bosco, *Securing the Sacred*.
31 Cf. Laustsen and Wæver, "In Defence of Religion," 708.
32 Ibid., 719. Carsten Bagge Lauststen and Ole Wæver are of the opinion that in the case of religion, faith becomes the referent object and the criterion for survival becomes being. This is contrasted with other referent objects investigated in the Copenhagen School such as states, nations, the environment, and firms whose four corresponding criteria of survival include sovereignty, identity, sustainability and avoiding bankruptcy. See Laustsen and Wæver, "In Defence of Religion," 718–719.
33 Cf. Keyes et al., "The Burden of Loss," 864–871.
34 Cf. Ruiz, "Personal Agency in Feminist Theory."
35 Cf. Krause, "Contested Questions, Current Trajectories."
36 Madhok et al., *Gender*, 4.

Works Cited

Bosco, Robert, *Securing the Sacred: Religion, National Security, and the Western State*, Michigan: University of Michigan Press, 2014.

Bramadat, Paul, "The Public, the Political and the Possible: Religion and Radicalization in Canada and Beyond," in *Religious Radicalization and Securitization in Canada and Beyond,* edited by Paul Bramadat and Lorne Dawson, Toronto: University of Toronto Press, 2014, 3–33.

Buzan, Barry, Ole Wæver, and Jaap de Wilde, *Security: A New Framework for Analysis*, London: Routledge, 1998.

Collins, Patricia, *Black Feminist Thought: Knowledge, Consciousness and the Politics of Empowerment*, New York: Routledge, 1998.
Collins, Patricia, *Black Sexual Politics: African Americans, Gender, and the New Racism*, New York: Routledge, 2004.
Gardiner, Judith Kegan, *Provoking Agents: Gender and Agency in Theory and Practice*, Urbana: University of Illinois Press, 1995.
Gunga, Samson, "The Politics of Widowhood and Re-Marriage among the Luo of Kenya," *Thought and Practice: A Journal of the Philosophical Association of Kenya* 1, 1 (2009): 161–174.
Keyes, Katherine, Charissa Pratt, Sandro Galea, Katie McLaughlin, Karestan Koenen, and Katherine Shear, "The Burden of Loss: Unexpected Death of a Loved One and Psychiatric Disorders Across the Life Course in a National Study," *American Journal of Psychiatry* 171 (2014): 864–871.
Krause, Sharon, "Contested Questions, Current Trajectories: Feminism in Political Theory Today," *Politics & Gender* 7, 1 (2011): 105–111.
Laustsen, Carsten Bagge and Ole Wæver, "In Defence of Religion: Sacred Referent: Objects for Securitization," *Millenium* 29, 3 (2000): 705–739.
Madhok, Sumi, Anne Phillips, and Kalpana Wilson (eds.), *Gender, Agency, and Coercion*, New York: Palgrave MacMillan, 2013.
Maseno, Loreen, "Securitizing Places of Worship in Kenya: The Case of Faith Evangelistic Ministry (FEM)," in *Religion and Human Security in Africa*, edited by Chitando, Ezra and Joram Tarusarira, New York: Routledge, 2019, 102–113.
Maseno-Ouma, Loreen, *How Abanyole African Widows Understand Christ: Explaining Redemption through the Propagation of Lineage*, New York: Edwin Mellen Press, 2014.
K'Olewe, Ochieng' O., "*Benga* and *Ohangla* Orature: The Subversive Traditional Curriculum," *Muziki* 10, 1 (2013), 33–49, https://doi.org/10.1080/18125980.2013.852742
Ocholla-Ayayo, Andrev, *Traditional Ideology and Ethics among the Southern Luo*, Uppsala: Scandinavian Institute of African Studies, 1976.
Odhiambo, Christopher and Loreen Maseno, "Dramatic Irony as an Intervention Strategy in Two Dholuo Films: Kalausi and The Cleansing," *Imbizo* 9, 2 (2019). https://doi.org/10.25159/2078-9785/5775
Ongati, Rose, "Recontextualization of *Orutu* Music of the Luo of Kenya: 1930 to 2006," Unpublished PhD Thesis, Maseno University, 2008.
Reuters Online Report. https://www.reuters.com/article/us-health-coronavirus-kenya-burial-prote-idUSKBN23J2X0
Ruiz, Maria, "Personal Agency in Feminist Theory: Evicting the Illusive Dweller," *The Behavior Analyst / MABA*, September (1998). https://doi.org/10.1007/BF03391962
Shiino, Wakana, "Death and Funeral Rituals Among the Luo in South Nyanza," *African Study Monographs* 18, 3, 4 (1997): 213–228.
Standard Newspaper Article. https://www.standardmedia.co.ke/nyanza/article/2001374833/police-probe-death-of-singer-abenny-jachiga.
Watson, Scott, "'Framing' the Copenhagen School: Integrating Literature on Threat Construction," *Millennium: Journal of International Studies* 40, 2 (2012): 279–301.
WHO 2020. https://covid19.who.int/region/afro/country/cf.
Youde, Jeremy, "Who's Afraid of a Chicken? Securitization and Avian Flu," *Democracy and Security* 4, 2 (2008): 148–169.

4 'He Has Filled the Hungry with Good Things' (Luke 1:53)

Theologizing on the Pandemic, *Pagpupuri*, and Pantries

Ma. Maricel S. Ibita and Ma. Marilou S. Ibita

1 Introduction

When the COVID-19 pandemic halted worldwide activities in March 2020, D. Kessler described the global emotion as micro-macro levels of grief because of the disruptions COVID-19 caused.[1] As insecurity sets in, A. Grant noticed that "languishing" became the "dominant emotion of 2021."[2] For Kessler, finding meaning helps to manage the grief that affected people feel, while Grant counseled that counting small victories like completing a small project, engaging in a meaningful conversation, or having a worthwhile goal transcends languishing.[3] In the pandemic's third year, a more basic need necessitates immediate response: global hunger. It counters the United Nations Sustainable Development Goal 2 of Zero Hunger by 2030. The World Food Program estimates that 811 million people go to bed hungry every night, with 48.9 million in emergency levels of hunger brought about by the multifaceted impacts of 4Cs – the COVID-19 pandemic, climate crisis, military conflicts, and the rising cost of reaching people in need.[4] To integrate these pandemic responses, we propose that theologizing on Mary's *Magnificat* (in Filipino, "*pagpupuri,*" "to praise") to the God who fills the hungry with good things (Luke 1:53) and on the catastrophic food insecurity that the 4Cs bring will allow individuals and communities to respond more effectively.

Our investigation employs the enhanced pastoral cycle of SEE-JUDGE-ACT-EVALUATE-CELEBRATE. This theory to praxis methodology originates from the SEE-JUDGE-ACT of Joseph Cardinal Cardijn who ministered to the young Christian workers and was affirmed in *Mater et Magistra* (236–237) as vital in living out the Catholic Social Teachings.[5] In Latin America, young Catholics expanded it with two more steps: EVALUATING the discerned action and CELEBRATING its result.[6] In theologizing about the pandemic, the *Magnificat/Pagpupuri,* and the pantries, we will locate Mary in the context of hunger in the Scriptures and 1st century CE Roman Palestine and relate her experiences to the context of Filipino urban poor women who opened community pantries to address the hunger due to the 4Cs. Next, we will analyze the relationship among hunger, Mary, Jesus and his meals in Luke, and the pandemic. We will then highlight the flourishing

DOI: 10.4324/b22930-5

community pantries in the Philippines as a communal ACTION against hunger and EVALUATE them in light of our socio-economic-political-theological analysis. Finally, we will underline the implication of this study in the CELEBRATION of the Eucharist as we build back better in a post-COVID-19 era guided by the United Nations Sustainable Goal of Zero Hunger (UNSDG#2).

2 See

Biblical references to famine, hunger, and malnutrition caused by soil infertility and climate change-induced droughts,[7] warfare, and God's judgment abound from Genesis to Revelation.[8] When hunger occurs, the poor are forced to sell their land and/or themselves as slaves (Amos 2:6–8). Women bear the hunger's brunt personally, like Ruth and the Zarephath widow (1 Kings 17:8–16). Famine exposes women like Sarah and Rebekah (Gen 12:10–20; 26:1–13) to gender violence. Inequality worsened when the monarchy institutionalized and supported latifundialization, the granting of land rights to their cohorts (Isaiah 5:8; Micah 2:1–2).[9] When cases of royal breach of the sacred result in plague or famine, the ancient peoples view these catastrophes as punishment from the deity and offer sacrifices to appease the gods and abate the disaster.[10] Since social structures should make sure that covenant life pervades society, the litmus test of obedience is abundance, while disobedience results in famine (Deut 28). Thus, solving hunger involves the individual (Job 31:16–17; Tobit 1:8, 17; 2:2), the leadership and societal structures, and ultimately, God (Isa 58; 65:21–22; Ps 33:18–19; 146:7).[11] Pervasive injustice leads to nutritional hunger and even to famine of God's word (Amos 8:11).[12]

As the aforementioned texts show, sometimes divine assistance against hunger has also been expressed by reversals like the song of Hannah in 1 Samuel 2:5: "Those who were full have hired themselves out for bread, but those who were hungry are fat with spoil."[13] Mary's *Magnificat* echoes Hannah's song (Luke 1:46–55, especially v. 53): "he has filled the hungry with good things, and sent the rich away empty." Against its socio-economic-political background, the *Magnificat* intensifies its revolutionary message. J.S. Kloppenborg's investigation of Jewish Palestine from the 3rd century BCE to the early 2nd century CE hints at a private farm tenancy system which led to agricultural exploitation through the growth of large estates, tenancy implementation, and shift from polyculture to export-oriented monoculture.[14] These practices resulted in underemployed laborers and 'free' tenants who became more exposed to hunger and more disadvantaged during famines, as pictured in the LXX, the parables of Jesus, and the Mishnah.[15] S. Friesen's 7-point poverty scale (PS) in the Roman empire during the time of Paul describes the imperial, regional, and municipal elites (PS 1–3, respectively), those with moderate surplus resources (PS 4), and the poor who had a stable life near subsistence, subsistence, and below subsistence levels (PS 5–7, respectively).[16] "Subsistence level" here is "the resources needed to procure enough calories in food to maintain the human body," the calorific needs necessary for a quality of life frequently shortened by chronic malnutrition and diseases.[17]

It seems that the world has not changed much since then. COVID-19, climate change, military conflicts, and the rising cost of sending food aid complicate and magnify hunger.[18] Worldwide, more people are dying from hunger than from COVID-19 infections because lockdowns caused massive job loss, compounded in some places by ecological emergencies and violent conflicts.[19] This situation is true in the Philippines because the government generally adopted a more militaristic than medical approach to the pandemic, resulting in "human rights violations, deterioration of social cohesion, health and vaccine concerns, and gender-based violations."[20] The Philippine hunger situation is more complex in areas of conflict and those devastated by natural hazards within the Pacific ring of fire like typhoons, flooding, and volcanic eruptions, which turn into disasters because of government's unpreparedness.[21] In the first six months of the COVID-19 lockdown, the Social Weather Stations recorded that involuntary hunger affected 7.6 million households severely ('often' or 'always' in the last quarter) and 2.2 million households moderately ('only once' or 'a few times' in the last quarter).[22]

Since the Philippines is a predominantly Christian nation, many of its inhabitants will ask the question: Does the Bible contain text traditions that help to discern effective responses to hunger when efforts from the government are lacking?

3 Judge

The God of the Bible reverses the politics of hunger.[23] Obedience to God's covenant brings flourishing because societal structures ensure that there is no poverty among the people, while communal generosity is supposed to support those who are impoverished by adversity (Deut 15:4–11). R.W. Klein accentuates the bifocal vision on hunger comprised by the need for salvation in the beatitudes for those who hunger and thirst for righteousness (Matt 5:6) and for the plain, earthy, caloric food found in the blessings to the hungry (Luke 6:21) and woes to those filled yet will go hungry (6:25).[24] Let us briefly investigate Luke's alimentary theology, which the *Magnificat* opens to us and guides us to Jesus' meal ministry.

Mary's *Magnificat* shows a *kairos* moment as she remembers the faithfulness of the Lord in the past and anticipates some of the themes of Jesus' ministry. L.E. Frizzell acknowledges that the *Magnificat* continues the women of prayers in the Hebrew Bible (Deborah, Hannah, Miriam) and the LXX (mother of the seven martyrs, Esther, Judith, Susanna) who were graced by God for the deliverance of the people.[25] With the other Lukan infancy canticles, Mary's song integrates the Jewish concepts of God's glory, blessing, mercy (*hesed*), faith, peace (*shalom*), and the prayers of the *Amidah*.[26] For S. Carruth, it reveals several unique Lukan themes that characterize Jesus' words and deeds: joy and salvation, prophecy, and prayer.[27] In this contribution, the *Magnificat* will serve as a foretaste of Jesus' meal ministry.

The *Magnificat* forms part of the infancy narrative in Luke (1:5–2:52). It binds the parallel annunciations to Zechariah (1:5–25) and Mary (1:26–38) and the parallel births of John the Baptist (1:57–80) and Jesus (2:1–21). Sandwiched by the temple events of Zechariah's incense offering (1:5–25) and the presentation of Jesus (2:22–28), it further solemnizes the infancy narrative. It also launches the series of canticles to the God of Israel and the fulfillment of the promised Messiah by Zechariah at the birth of John, by the angels at Jesus' birth, and by Simeon and Anna at Jesus' circumcision. The collective hopes of Israel in these stories are the backdrops of Jesus' future meal ministry, prophesied in Mary's song: "he has filled the hungry with good things, and sent the rich away empty" (1:53).

Within its larger literary context, the *Magnificat* foreshadows who and how Jesus will be. M. Ibita previously noted a Christological understanding of Jesus as guest, host, and servant at table in Luke.[28] We will contextualize these titles of Jesus from the lens of the Magnificat's food reference.

The same Spirit that overshadowed Mary in the Annunciation filled Elizabeth to exclaim how blessed Mary and the fruit of her womb are (Luke 1:41–42). In response, Mary's spirit magnified the Lord and her soul rejoiced in God, her Savior, indicating the communal identity of the divine for Israel and Mary's own saving experience of the Lord as God of reversal. Her song "he has filled the hungry with good things, and sent the rich away empty" (1:53), proleptically speaks of the hunger and food motif in Jesus' ministry.

The Holy Spirit led Jesus to the desert; there, Jesus fasted for 40 days and withstood the temptations of the devil (4:1–4). In his mission inaugural, Jesus cited Isaiah with a one-liner commentary, "Today this scripture has been fulfilled in your hearing" (4:21), which sparked amazement and disagreement. Jesus' reply that no prophet is accepted in one's hometown referred to Elijah's encounter with the widow of Zarephath during the severe famine of three years and six months resulted in violence which endangered Jesus (4:16–30).

In his Galilean ministry (4:16–9:51), Jesus, his disciples, tax collectors, and others started as guests of Levi (5:27–39). Jesus was Simon's guest when an unwelcomed woman anointed him (7:36–50). The Galilean ministry closes with a shift in Jesus' role from guest to being the host, along with his apostles, when he fed the crowd (9:10–17).

During his Jerusalem journey (9:51-19:27), Jesus was mainly a guest of different hosts. Martha welcomed and served (διακονεῖν) him (10:38–42). Then, Jesus, though a guest in an unnamed Pharisee's house (11:37–54), spewed woes to remind those around him about more important matters, making the scribes and the Pharisees who were also there very hostile against him (11:53). According to Luke 14:1–24, Jesus attended a Sabbath meal in a house of a ruler who was a Pharisee when he healed a man with dropsy, gave a lesson on humility, and told a parable on a banquet and invited guests. Before reaching Jerusalem, Jesus dined with Zacchaeus, the chief tax collector

(19:1–10). In his Galilean ministry and journey to Jerusalem, Jesus provided nourishment for both body and spirit. Those who were open were filled with nutritional and spiritual food, while those who were not ended up being empty of his teachings and filled with rancor against him.

In Jerusalem (19:28-23:56), Jesus's ministry shifted from guest to host and even servant at the Passover meal before his passion and death (22:14–38, especially vv. 15, 27). In Jesus' parting words and action with request for remembering, he identified himself with the bread and cup of wine (22:19–20). These various roles of being guest, host, and servant once again happened at Emmaus post-resurrection when the two disciples finally recognized the Risen Jesus in the breaking of the bread (24:13–35). In meeting the other disciples, the resurrected Jesus proved his identity by requesting for something to eat which they answered by giving him broiled fish (24:41–42). Thus, Jesus' mission which began with fasting ended and was completed with him requesting food. Jesus' meal ministry is tied to his evolving identity as guest, host, food and drink, and servant at table depending on the changing contexts.

This meal ministry of Jesus inspires and mirrors the hunger response of Christians during the pandemic in the Philippines. Even before hunger peaked in September 2020 and face-to-face Eucharistic gatherings were prohibited, a lot of churches became relief preparation venues for assembling food packs and health kits, temporary accommodations for those stranded by the lockdowns, and centers for psychological first aid.[29] Our educational institutions like the Ateneo de Manila University (AdMU) and the De La Salle University (DLSU) also became temporary shelters for medical frontliners and the homeless, providing them with warm meals, food packs, and safety kits while also offering the school community with financial aids, psycho-spiritual care, and other ways to help each other.[30] These are institutional responses. How did the marginalized, especially the women, respond to the hunger brought about by the 4Cs?

4 Act

While the COVID-19 pandemic affected everyone, the poor suffered most of its effects. E. Tadem surveyed five grassroots cases in poverty-stricken urban areas and indigenous communities.[31] He found out that in these marginalized communities, "principles of solidarity, social cohesion, organizational fitness, and sharing" offered minimum relief measures. Nevertheless, due to the militarized approach, basic public services were lacking, livelihood opportunities were scarce, the government's intensified social amelioration program (SAP) was unreliable, and their community resources were limited, so they could not fully respond to the pandemic-related concerns of their members.[32] For women, immediate areas of concern heightened by the quarantine levels include economic shock, sexual violence inside and outside their homes, and limited access to quality online education for children.[33]

Given these realities, women in grassroots communities took upon themselves how they could respond to the COVID-19 challenges together. During the height of the COVID-19 lockdown, our Vincentian missionary friend, D.F. Pilario, Dean of St. Vincent School of Theology, and his community used to go out daily to deliver food packs to street dwellers while ministering to the families in their mission parish at the garbage dump of Payatas, Quezon City. As help from the government and non-government organizations were wanting, the women themselves started urban gardening because their husbands lost their jobs and their families were hungry. In his lecture on "Surviving the Pandemic: Solidarity in the Margins" last December 6, 2021 at St. John's University, New York, Pilario recounted,

> After three months of relief distribution, we gathered to assess what we were doing. I asked, 'After three months and with all of the risks involved, what made you stay? Why are you still here?' Their response was, 'In the Bible, Jesus asked us to feed the hungry. How can we stay safe at home when our neighbor is dying? How can we sleep when our neighbor is hungry?[34]

The same experience was narrated by the Alliance of Peoples' Organizations Along the Manggahan Floodway (APOAMF) in our multi-sectoral, interdisciplinary, and international community research called Urban Poor Women and Children with Academics for Reaching and Delivering on UNSDGs in the Philippines (UPWARD-UP).[35] The leaders themselves, mostly women, planned the health protocols, gave monetary and food assistance to those who were infected, cooperated with government offices for their housing, water, and sanitation issues to better manage COVID-19, started urban gardening, and supported the online sale of viands to augment family's nutritional and economic needs. They also caught on the viral idea of erecting community pantries. What is this?

J. Suazo tells this story, which inspired the whole country.[36] Ana Patricia Non owns a furniture refurbishing business that hired workers severely affected by the pandemic. As she found it difficult to make ends meet, she thought of others who were in a worse situation, such as the daily wage earners. She looked for a frequently visited place in the community and approached the owners of a convenience store to inquire if she could use their front space for opening a community pantry. With their approval, she rushed home to get her prepared bamboo cart with rice, vegetables, milk, vitamins, canned goods, soap, and other essentials and brought them at that accessible place to service nearby villages. Thus, she launched the Maginhawa Community Pantry and posted it on her Facebook account. After a few hours, family and friends sent cash donations which Non used to buy replenishments for the next day. Within 24 hours, her post became viral and other Filipinos reached out to help. Non encouraged those outside the radius of Maginhawa

Community Pantry to start their own.[37] Soon several community pantries sprouted around the metropolis and nationwide.

Non started the community pantry on April 14, 2021 at Maginhawa because "I am tired of complaining, of inaction [of the government]."[38] The initiative's basic principle is "From each according to one's ability, to each according to one's needs," which her sister translated as "*Magbigay ayon sa kakayahan, kumuha batay sa pangangailangan.*" This principle mirrors Acts 2:44–45; 4:34, according to which the early Christian communities shared their belongings so that there was no needy person among them.

The community pantries idea took on many forms: halal foods for Muslim communities, kitchen staples, pet foods, garden materials, toys, books, and even contraceptives for sexual health, and some with an eco-friendly note of BYOB ("bring your own bag/bottles").[39] Some sourced their donations from local farmers' organizations to help them sell their produce.[40] By August 2021, there were over 6,700 community pantries nationwide and to sustain them, an adopt-a-community-pantry initiative was supported by the two leading Catholic universities in the country, AdMU and DLSU.[41]

The community pantries also involved those that urban society usually shun, like the indigenous peoples.[42] When they heard about the Maginhawa community pantry and as a thanksgiving for supermarket goods donations they received, some indigenous peoples from the nearby Rizal province thought of gifting their farm products to urban poor communities who were experiencing hunger the most. Despite suffering from the losses of ecotourism due to the lockdowns and threatened by the government's Kaliwa dam project, which they are protesting against, Renato Ibanez, leader of Dumagat Remontado group SUKATAN-LN, wisely said that the pantry initiative unites rural and urban Filipinos. "[W]ith this food, all of us in this country are eating as one – we're not divided, we're not fighting, we're all dining at one table."[43]

5 Evaluate

While many were impressed by the community pantries, some were skeptical and even antagonistic. Suazo noted that volunteers were able to realize how they could contribute to the community, which shows the best of humanity in the worst of times. While some questioned its sustainability, the pantry initiators were surprised that people also reached out offering their help. While some were concerned about people hoarding goods, volunteers said that beneficiaries discerned first what they really need and only got enough, ensuring goods for others.[44] For Non, those who returned for more means that they really needed supplies. She underlined that the pantries were not permanent solutions but they can tide people over to survive the complexities of the pandemic. While people hailed the pantries as a solidarity movement and a show of Filipino resiliency, Non was also realistic in saying that it was a response and unity born out of necessity.[45] She underlined that community building takes baby steps and that everyone must learn how to share, not just goods but also efforts and time in repacking the goods, making sure that residents observed health protocols. People resonated and replicated the pantries because it is closest to the most basic of needs, a hungry stomach.[46]

For sociologist A.C. Presto, the community pantries can be understood not as charity but mutual aid during this crisis and also as acts of resistance "first, against a government that fails to adequately address citizens' needs; second, against a biased and discriminatory view of the poor as selfish and greedy; and third, against aid initiatives from institutions that are difficult to trust."[47] Notably, the supporters of the pantries include the poor themselves, from farmers who shared their produce to tricycle drivers who volunteered to repack donations, dispelling the idea that only the rich can donate and that the poor are greedy.[48]

Unfortunately, the pantries have been weaponized. M. Andrada, a popular culture expert and professor of Philippine studies, remarks that the use of cardboard boxes as signboards symbolizes three different things: used as containers of goods and signages of the pantries, they are very practical and the poor can easily relate with its everyday use; they have also been utilized by advocacy groups in demonstrations to express their aspirations, grievances, and demands against the rising inequality and poverty; and while these cardboards have been used to mark the victims of the highly criticized extrajudicial killing in the Duterte government's fight against illegal drugs which is presently being investigated by the International Criminal Court, [49] the cardboards now signifies food for the hungry and solidarity with those who suffer most.[50]

For these reasons, Non was called Satan and the community pantries were "red-tagged" or identified as communist by the government's anti-insurgency spokespersons, Lt. Gen. A. Parlade, Jr. and Undersecretary L. Badoy.[51] National Privacy Commissioner R.E. Liboro denounced and urged them to stop profiling and red-tagging pandemic heroes.[52] While these irresponsible and dangerous comments stalled Non's community pantry for a while, citizens were quick to defend her against Parlade and Badoy while calling for protection of community pantries.[53] In response, Vice President Leni Robredo defended Non, some senators threatened to defund the anti-insurgency group, the National Security Adviser ordered Parlade and Badoy to desist in making statements against community pantries, the Department of Interior and Local Government (DILG) conceded that the police should not question the pantry organizers, and with the Metro Manila Development Authority, they suggested that organizers should first coordinate with village officials about their initiatives.[54] Non's mother, Zena Bernardo, asked the Ombudsman to suspend and to hold Badoy responsible as her

> acts of red-tagging and disseminating false information and fake news online and offline against community pantries and the organizers thereof constitute disinformation, abuse and misuse of official authority

> and public resources, and worse, endangerment of the lives and safety [of] ordinary citizens.[55]

With this dialogue between the *Magnificat* and the community pantries filling of the hungry amidst the 4Cs, salvation

> goes beyond the interior and personal to the communal and even the political. It is, in fact, the undoing of ways of thinking and of economic, social, and political systems and policies that result in poverty, hunger, and status distinctions.[56]

As Helder Camara said, "When I feed the poor, they call me a saint, but when I ask why the poor have no food, they call me a Communist."[57]

6 Celebrate

Pilario asks, "How does our theology of the Eucharist take into account this experience of hunger by millions of our people?"[58] Our investigation shows that hunger for nutritional food (Luke 6:21) must be correlated to hunger for righteousness (Matt 5:6), that feeding the hungry and asking why there is hunger are necessary acts of mercy and mission of all Christians. As the Eucharist remembers Jesus' meal ministry where he was guest, host, servant, and food for the journey, we must re-live it today and extend it from the liturgical celebration to the community, just like the Payatas and APOAMF women and the pantries inspired by Non. These efforts embody Hannah's song and Mary's *Magnificat* in *full,* which praise the God who fills the hungry with good things.

7 Conclusion and Implication

As a social document,[59] the *Magnificat* invites us to a whole new, different world view of being communities steeped in God, in history, and how God empowers us to be agents of salvation in realizing the Zero Hunger UNSDG. Using the enhanced pastoral spiral of SEE-JUDGE-ACT-EVALUATE-CELEBRATE, we theologized on Mary's *Magnificat* and the socio-economic-political-religious aspects of hunger in the Bible and Jesus' meal ministry under the Roman Empire, which has similarities with the 4Cs of today's hunger: COVID-19 pandemic, climate change, military conflicts, and the rising cost of sending food aid. Mary's *Magnificat* welcomes us to the meal ministry of Jesus as guest, host, servant, and food in Luke. This theologizing enriches our meaning-making and recognizes the winning moments of Filipino women in urban poor communities of Payatas and APOAMF to address hunger, including Non's inspiring community pantry story. In Hannah's and Mary's songs, feeding the hungry is prophetic and subversive. The Spirit of the God of reversal in the *Magnificat* impels us to be like Mary who went in haste to help others, graced to embody and give birth to Jesus – the guest, host, servant, and food and drink – again and again during the pandemic and beyond.

8 Concise Summary/Future Research

The Theologizing on the Pandemic, *Pagpupuri,* and Pantries demonstrated how the enhanced pastoral cycle of SEE-JUDGE-ACT-EVALUATE-CELEBRATE is a valuable method of theologizing itself. It can be employed to engage other social issues with the help of the Bible to provide new insights and new research directions. This way of engaging Mary's *Magnificat* opens up new inquiries about a gendered look at hunger, how hunger affects women in the Bible nutritionally, and in connection with hunger-related experiences of gendered violence. Consequently, the biblical theologizing will help churches to respond to current problems, which will have an impact on Mariology, Christology, Ecclesiology, and Liturgy. Finally, these enriched theological reflections can further help discover the oft-neglected inspiration of religious traditions and the oft-overlooked force of religious groups and religion itself as vital resources in achieving the UNSDGs, especially UNSDG 2: Zero Hunger.

Notes

1 Scott Berinato, "That Discomfort You're Feeling Is Grief," *Harvard Business Review*, 23 March 2020, https://hbr.org/2020/03/that-discomfort-youre-feeling-is-grief.
2 Adam Grant, "There's a Name for the Blah You're Feeling: It's Called Languishing," *The New York Times*, 19 April 2021, https://www.nytimes.com/2021/04/19/well/mind/covid-mental-health-languishing.html.
3 Berinato, "Discomfort"; Grant, "Name."
4 World Food Program, "A Hunger Catastrophe: Marching towards Starvation," *www.wfp.Org*, n.d., https://www.wfp.org/hunger-catastrophe.
5 See Justin Sands, "Introducing Cardinal Cardijn's See–Judge–Act as an Interdisciplinary Method to Move Theory into Practice," *Religions* 9.4, 129 (2018): 3/10, https://doi.org/10.3390/rel9040129; Daniel Franklin Pilario, "Revisiting See-Judge-Act: Reflections from Asia," *Concilium* 1 (2016): 83.
6 See Ma. Marilou Ibita, "Meals and Mission: A Contextual Reading of the Lukan Meal Scenes in the Filipino Context," in *A Flourishing Faith: Celebrating 500 Years of Christianity in the Philippines*, ed. Fides del Castillo (Paranaque, Philippines: Don Bosco School of Theology, 2021), 47–70.
7 Eric H. Cline, "Climate Change Doomed the Ancients," *The New York Times*, 27 May 2014, http://www.nytimes.com/2014/05/28/opinion/climate-change-doomed-the-ancients.html.
8 See Ralph W. Klein, "The God of the Bible Confronts the Politics of Hunger," *CurTM* 17.2 (1990): 110–117.
9 See Klein, "God," 112.
10 See K. C. Hanson, "When the King Crosses the Line: Royal Deviance and Restitution in Levantine Ideologies," *BTB* 26.1 (1996): 11–25, https://doi.org/10.1177/014610799602600103.
11 Klein, "God," 112–114.
12 Klein, "God," 114.

13 Unless otherwise indicated, our study uses the *New Revised Standard Version Bible* (New York, NY: Division of Christian Education of the National Council of the Churches of Christ in the United States of America, 1989), BibleWorks, v.9.
14 John S. Kloppenborg, "The Growth and Impact of Agricultural Tenancy in Jewish Palestine (III BCE-I CE)," *JESHO* 51.1 (2008): 31–66, https://doi.org/10.1163/156852008X287549.
15 Kloppenborg, "Growth," 31–66.
16 Steven J. Friesen, "Poverty in Pauline Studies: Beyond the So-Called New Consensus," *JSNT* 26.3 (2004): 341.
17 Friesen, "Poverty," 343.
18 World Food Program, "Hunger."
19 Abdul Rahaman et al., "The Increasing Hunger Concern and Current Need in the Development of Sustainable Food Security in the Developing Countries," *Trends in Food Science & Technology* 113 (2021): 423–429, https://doi.org/10.1016/j.tifs.2021.04.048.
20 Nick Aspinwall, "As Hunger Rises, Philippine Authorities Take Aim at Critics," *The New Humanitarian*, 20 April 2021, https://www.thenewhumanitarian.org/news/2021/4/20/food-hunger-and-covid-19-in-the-philippines; Ditte Fallesen, "How COVID-19 Impacted Vulnerable Communities in the Philippines," *World Bank Blogs*, 10 November 2021, https://blogs.worldbank.org/eastasiapacific/how-covid-19-impacted-vulnerable-communities-philippines.
21 See World Food Program, *Typhoon Rolly and Typhoon Ulysses*, Situation Report #6, March 22, 2021, https://reliefweb.int/report/philippines/typhoon-rolly-and-typhoon-ulysses-situation-report-6–22-march-2021.
22 Social Weather Stations, "SWS September 17–20, 2020 National Mobile Phone Survey – Report No. 2: Hunger at New Record-High 30.7% of Families," *Social Weather Stations*, 27 September 2020, https://www.sws.org.ph/swsmain/artcldisppage/?artcsyscode=ART-20200927135430.
23 Klein, "God," 114.
24 Klein, "God," 114.
25 Lawrence E Frizzell, "Mary and the Biblical Heritage," *Marian Studies* 46 (1995): 26–40.
26 Lawrence E. Frizzell, "Mary's Magnificat: Sources and Themes," *Marian Studies* 50.1 (1999): 38–59.
27 Shawn Carruth, "A Song of Salvation: The Magnificat, Luke 1:46–55," *TBT* 50.6 (2012): 345–349.
28 Ma. Marilou Ibita, "Dining with Jesus in the Third Gospel: Celebrating Eucharist in the Third World," *East Asian Pastoral Review* 42.3 (2005), http://www.eapi.org.ph/resources/eapr/east-asian-pastoral-review-2005/volume-42–2005-number-3/dining-with-jesus-in-the-third-gospel-celebrating-eucharist-in-the-third-world/.
29 See Joseph Peter Calleja, "Philippine Govt Praises Church Pandemic Efforts," *UCANews.Com*, 29 April 2020, https://www.ucanews.com/news/philippine-govt-praises-church-pandemic-efforts/87859.
30 Angela Maree Encomienda, "A Caring Community Is a Healthy Community: LS Cura Project," *Ateneo de Manila University*, 14 September 2021, https://2012.ateneo.edu/ls/loyola-schools/news/features/caring-community-healthy-community-ls-cura-project. For a more complete listing of pandemic initiatives at De la Salle University, see https://www.dlsu.edu.ph/covid19initiatives/
31 Eduardo C. Tadem, "How the Marginalized Fight Their Way Through the Pandemic: The Philippine Case," *UNESCO Inclusive Policy Lab*, 22 January 2021, https://en.unesco.org/inclusivepolicylab/analytics/how-marginalized-fight-their-way-through-pandemic-philippine-case.
32 Tadem, "Marginalized."

33 Akanksha Khullar, "COVID-19: Impact on Women in the Philippines," *ReliefWeb*, 27 September 2021, https://reliefweb.int/report/philippines/covid-19-impact-women-philippines.
34 "Combating Hunger Amidst COVID-19 in the Philippines," *www.st.johns.edu*, 9 December 2021, https://www.stjohns.edu/about/news/2021-12-09/combating-hunger-amidst-covid-19-philippines.
35 The South Initiative program of VLIR-UOS, Belgium funds this PH2020-SIN294A101 project. It involves the Katholieke Universiteit Leuven in Belgium, the Ateneo de Manila University, the St. Vincent School of Theology of Adamson University, and the De la Salle University in the Philippines. We work with our non-government organization partner Community Organizers Multiversity (COM) which assists the Alliance of Peoples' Organizations along the Manggahan Floodway (APOAMF) in Pasig City, Philippines in their urban poor advocacies.
36 Juli Suazo, "What the Community Pantry Movement Means for Filipinos," *www.cnnphilippines.Com*, 19 April 2021, https://www.cnnphilippines.com/life/culture/2021/4/19/community-pantry-filipinos-pandemic.html.
37 Suazo, "Community."
38 Iya Gozum, "'*Pagod Na Ako Sa* Inaction': How a Community Pantry Rose to Fill Gaps in Gov't Response," *rappler.com*, 17 April 2021, https://www.rappler.com/moveph/community-pantry-covid-19-lockdown-april-2021/.
39 Diana G. Mendoza, "'Hope in the Darkest of Times,'" *www.pacificislandtimes.com*, 19 April 2021, https://www.pacificislandtimes.com/post/hope-in-the-darkest-of-times; Brooke Villanueva, "Contraceptives, Toys, Pet Food, Zero Waste, and Other Unique PH Community Pantries," *www.philstarlife.com*, 23 April 2021, https://philstarlife.com/news-and-views/148254-unique-ph-community-pantries.
40 Suazo, "Community."
41 Patricia B. Mirason, "Adopt-a-Community-Pantry Initiative Launched," *BusinessWorld Online*, 23 August 2021, https://www.bworldonline.com/the-nation/2021/08/23/390933/adopt-a-community-pantry-initiative-launched/.
42 Maverick Flores, "'*Isang Hapag-Kainan*': IPs and Community Pantries Work Together to Feed Cities," *rappler.com*, 30 May 2021, https://www.rappler.com/moveph/indigenous-people-community-pantries-work-together-feed-cities/.
43 Flores, "'*Isang Hapag-Kainan*.'"
44 Suazo, "Community."
45 Suazo, "Community."
46 Gozum, "*Pagod*."
47 Nikka G. Valenzuela, "Community Pantry: 'Not Charity, but Mutual Aid,'" *Inquirer.net*, 18 April 2021, https://newsinfo.inquirer.net/1420463/community-pantry-not-charity-but-mutual-aid.
48 Valenzuela, "Community.'"
49 Al Jazeera, "ICC Prosecutor to Reopen Philippines 'Drug War' Investigation," *Aljazeera.com*, 24 June 2022, https://www.aljazeera.com/news/2022/6/24/icc-prosecutor-plans-to-reopen-philippines-drug-war-investigation.
50 Marc Jayson Cayabyab, "Very Relatable: Analysts Believe Carton Signs, Basic Goods Make Community Pantries A Hit Among the Masses," *OneNews.Ph*, 21 April 2021, https://www.onenews.ph/articles/very-relatable-analysts-believe-carton-signs-basic-goods-make-community-pantries-a-hit-among-the-masses.
51 Catalina Ricci S. Madarang, "'Unnecessary, Unjust': Parlade Blasted for Comparing Maginhawa Pantry Organizer to Satan," *Interaksyon*, 22 April 2021, https://interaksyon.philstar.com/trends-spotlights/2021/04/22/190304/unnecessary-parlade-blasted-for-satan-reference-to-maginhawa-pantry-organizer/.
52 Madarang, "'Unnecessary."

53 Catalina Ricci S. Madarang, "Calls to 'Protect Community Pantries' Grow as Red Tagging Fears Halt Maginhawa Effort," *Interaksyon*, 20 April 2021, https://interaksyon.philstar.com/trends-spotlights/2021/04/20/190070/calls-for-protect-community-pantries-grow-as-red-tag-fears-temporarily-halt-maginhawa-community-pantry/.
54 Wendell Vigilia et al., "Leni Tells Gov't: Stop Witch-Hunt on Community Pantry Org," *www.malaya.com.ph*, 26 April 2021, https://malaya.com.ph/news_news/leni-tells-govt-stop-witch-hunt-on-community-pantry-organizers/.
55 Hanna Bordey, "Ombudsman Asked to Suspend, Hold Badoy Criminally Liable for Red-Tagging Patreng Non," *GMA News Online*, 13 April 2022, https://www.gmanetwork.com/news/topstories/nation/828419/ombudsman-asked-to-suspend-hold-badoy-criminally-liable-for-red-tagging-patreng-non/story/.
56 Carruth, "Song," 348.
57 Bernard Evans, "Archbishop Hélder Câmara, the People's Pastor, Shows Us How to Live," *U.S. Catholic*, 26 October 2020, https://uscatholic.org/articles/202010/archbishop-helder-camara-the-peoples-pastor-shows-us-another-way-to-live/.
58 "Combating."
59 Susan Connelly, "The Magnificat as Social Document," *Compass* 48.4 (2014): 8–11.

Works Cited

Al Jazeera, "ICC Prosecutor to Reopen Philippines 'Drug War' Investigation," *Aljazeera.Com*, 24 June 2022, https://www.aljazeera.com/news/2022/6/24/icc-prosecutor-plans-to-reopen-philippines-drug-war-investigation.

Aspinwall, Nick, "As Hunger Rises, Philippine Authorities Take Aim at Critics," *The New Humanitarian*, 20 April 2021, https://www.thenewhumanitarian.org/news/2021/4/20/food-hunger-and-covid-19-in-the-philippines.

Berinato, Scott, "That Discomfort You're Feeling Is Grief," *Harvard Business Review*, 23 March 2020, https://hbr.org/2020/03/that-discomfort-youre-feeling-is-grief.

Bordey, Hanna, "Ombudsman Asked to Suspend, Hold Badoy Criminally Liable for Red-Tagging Patreng Non," *GMA News Online*, 13 April 2022, https://www.gmanetwork.com/news/topstories/nation/828419/ombudsman-asked-to-suspend-hold-badoy-criminally-liable-for-red-tagging-patreng-non/story/.

Calleja, Joseph Peter, "Philippine Govt Praises Church Pandemic Efforts," *UCANews.com*, 29 April 2020, https://www.ucanews.com/news/philippine-govt-praises-church-pandemic-efforts/87859.

Carruth, Shawn, "A Song of Salvation: The Magnificat, Luke 1:46–55," *TBT* 50.6 (2012): 345–349.

Cayabyab, Marc Jayson, "Very Relatable: Analysts Believe Carton Signs, Basic Goods Make Community Pantries a Hit Among the Masses," *OneNews.Ph*, 21 April 2021, https://www.onenews.ph/articles/very-relatable-analysts-believe-carton-signs-basic-goods-make-community-pantries-a-hit-among-the-masses.

Cline, Eric H., "Climate Change Doomed the Ancients," *The New York Times*, 27 May 2014, http://www.nytimes.com/2014/05/28/opinion/climate-change-doomed-the-ancients.html.

"Combating Hunger Amidst COVID-19 in the Philippines," *www.st.johns.edu*, 9 December 2021, https://www.stjohns.edu/about/news/2021-12-09/combating-hunger-amidst-covid-19-philippines.

Connelly, Susan, "The Magnificat as Social Document," *Compass* 48.4 (2014): 8–11.

Encomienda, Angela Maree, "A Caring Community Is a Healthy Community: LS Cura Project," *Ateneo de Manila University*, 14 September 2021, https://2012.ateneo.edu/ls/loyola-schools/news/features/caring-community-healthy-community-ls-cura-project.

Evans, Bernard, "Archbishop Hélder Câmara, the People's Pastor, Shows Us How to Live - U.S. Catholic." *U.S. Catholic*, 26 October 2020. - U.S. Catholic," *U.S. Catholic*, 26 October 2020, https://uscatholic.org/articles/202010/archbishop-helder-camara-the-peoples-pastor-shows-us-another-way-to-live/.

Fallesen, Ditte, "How COVID-19 Impacted Vulnerable Communities in the Philippines," *World Bank Blogs*, 10 November 2021, https://blogs.worldbank.org/eastasiapacific/how-covid-19-impacted-vulnerable-communities-philippines.

Flores, Maverick, "'*Isang Hapag-Kainan*': IPs and Community Pantries Work Together to Feed Cities," *rappler.com*, 30 May 2021, https://www.rappler.com/moveph/indigenous-people-community-pantries-work-together-feed-cities/.

Friesen, Steven J., "Poverty in Pauline Studies: Beyond the So-Called New Consensus," *JSNT* 26.3 (2004): 323–361.

Frizzell, Lawrence E., "Mary and the Biblical Heritage," *Marian Studies* 46 (1995): 26–40.

———, "Mary's Magnificat: Sources and Themes," *Marian Studies* 50.1 (1999): 38–59.

Gozum, Iya, "'*Pagod Na Ako Sa* Inaction': How a Community Pantry Rose to Fill Gaps in Gov't Response," *rappler.com*, 17 April 2021, https://www.rappler.com/moveph/community-pantry-covid-19-lockdown-april-2021/.

Grant, Adam, "There's a Name for the Blah You're Feeling: It's Called Languishing," *The New York Times*, 19 April 2021, https://www.nytimes.com/2021/04/19/well/mind/covid-mental-health-languishing.html.

Hanson, K. C., "When the King Crosses the Line: Royal Deviance and Restitution in Levantine Ideologies," *BTB* 26.1 (1996): 11–25, https://doi.org/10.1177/014610799602600103.

Ibita, Ma. Marilou, "Dining with Jesus in the Third Gospel: Celebrating Eucharist in the Third World," *East Asian Pastoral Review* 42.3 (2005), http://www.eapi.org.ph/resources/eapr/east-asian-pastoral-review-2005/volume-42-2005-number-3/dining-with-jesus-in-the-third-gospel-celebrating-eucharist-in-the-third-world/.

———, "Meals and Mission: A Contextual Reading of the Lukan Meal Scenes in the Filipino Context," in *A Flourishing Faith: Celebrating 500 Years of Christianity in the Philippines*, edited by Fides del Castillo, Paranaque, Philippines: Don Bosco School of Theology, 2021, 47–70.

Khullar, Akanksha, "COVID-19: Impact on Women in the Philippines," *ReliefWeb*, 27 September 2021, https://reliefweb.int/report/philippines/covid-19-impact-women-philippines.

Klein, Ralph W., "The God of the Bible Confronts the Politics of Hunger," *CurTM* 17.2 (1990): 110–117.

Kloppenborg, John S., "The Growth and Impact of Agricultural Tenancy in Jewish Palestine (III BCE-I CE)," *JESHO* 51.1 (2008): 31–66, https://doi.org/10.1163/156852008X287549.

Madarang, Catalina Ricci S., "Calls to 'Protect Community Pantries' Grow as Red Tagging Fears Halt Maginhawa Effort," *Interaksyon*, 20 April 2021, https://interaksyon.philstar.com/trends-spotlights/2021/04/20/190070/calls-for-protect-community-pantries-grow-as-red-tag-fears-temporarily-halt-maginhawa-community-pantry/.

———, "'Unnecessary, Unjust': Parlade Blasted for Comparing Maginhawa Pantry Organizer to Satan," *Interaksyon*, 22 April 2021, https://interaksyon.philstar.com/trends-spotlights/2021/04/22/190304/unnecessary-parlade-blasted-for-satan-reference-to-maginhawa-pantry-organizer/.

Mendoza, Diana G., "'Hope in the Darkest of Times,'" *www.pacificislandtimes.com*, 19 April 2021, https://www.pacificislandtimes.com/post/hope-in-the-darkest-of-times.

Mirason, Patricia B., "Adopt-a-Community-Pantry Initiative Launched," *BusinessWorld Online*, 23 August 2021, https://www.bworldonline.com/the-nation/2021/08/23/390933/adopt-a-community-pantry-initiative-launched/.

Pilario, Daniel Franklin, "Revisiting See-Judge-Act: Reflections from Asia," *Concilium* 1 (2016): 83–92.

Rahaman, Abdul, Ankita Kumari, Xin-An Zeng, Ibrahim Khalifa, Muhammad Adil Farooq, Narpinder Singh, Shahid Ali, Mahafooj Alee, and Rana Muhammad Aadil, "The Increasing Hunger Concern and Current Need in the Development of Sustainable Food Security in the Developing Countries," *Trends in Food Science & Technology* 113 (2021): 423–429, https://doi.org/10.1016/j.tifs.2021.04.048.

Sands, Justin, "Introducing Cardinal Cardijn's See–Judge–Act as an Interdisciplinary Method to Move Theory into Practice," *Religions* 9.4, 129 (2018): 10 pages, https://doi.org/10.3390/rel9040129.

Social Weather Stations, "SWS September 17–20, 2020 National Mobile Phone Survey – Report No. 2: Hunger at New Record-High 30.7% of Families," *Social Weather Stations*, 27 September 2020, https://www.sws.org.ph/swsmain/artcldisppage/?artcsyscode=ART-20200927135430.

Suazo, Juli, "What the Community Pantry Movement Means for Filipinos," *www.cnnphilippines.com*, 19 April 2021, https://www.cnnphilippines.com/life/culture/2021/4/19/community-pantry-filipinos-pandemic.html.

Tadem, Eduardo C., "How the Marginalized Fight Their Way Through the Pandemic: The Philippine Case," *UNESCO Inclusive Policy Lab*, 22 January 2021, https://en.unesco.org/inclusivepolicylab/analytics/how-marginalized-fight-their-way-through-pandemic-philippine-case.

Valenzuela, Nikka G., "Community Pantry: 'Not Charity, but Mutual Aid,'" *inquirer.net*, 18 April 2021, https://newsinfo.inquirer.net/1420463/community-pantry-not-charity-but-mutual-aid.

Vigilia, Wendell, Jocelyn Montemayor, Victor Reyes, and Noel Talacay, "Leni Tells Gov't: Stop Witch-Hunt on Community Pantry Org," *www.malaya.com.ph*, 25 April 2021, https://malaya.com.ph/news_news/leni-tells-govt-stop-witch-hunt-on-community-pantry-organizers/.

Villanueva, Brooke, "Contraceptives, Toys, Pet Food, Zero Waste, and Other Unique PH Community Pantries," *www.philstarlife.com*, 23 April 2021, https://philstarlife.com/news-and-views/148254-unique-ph-community-pantries.

World Food Program, "A Hunger Catastrophe: Marching towards Starvation," *www.wfp.org*, n.d., https://www.wfp.org/hunger-catastrophe.

———, *Typhoon Rolly and Typhoon Ulysses*, Situation Report #6, March 22, 2021, https://reliefweb.int/report/philippines/typhoon-rolly-and-typhoon-ulysses-situation-report-6-22-march-2021.

Part II

Rituals in Times of Trouble

5 Diseased Rites

Magic Tantras and Inflicted Illness

Aaron Michael Ullrey

1 Introduction

The COVID-19 pandemic has revealed varied cultural anxieties and universal human anxieties about disease and health. As this pandemic rages (and seems to be with us forever), those living through it must ask what counts as disease and what counts as health; when a pandemic lingers, as this one has, such concerns also linger. Is health freedom from general disease or is it freedom from a specific disease? Or is health the resolution and recovery from a disease? Or is health immunity to a disease (an immunity evasive to efforts against COVID-19)? Such concerns are not new—many traditions of Hinduism, or Hinduisms, conceive health and disease differently than modern, materialist worldviews.[1] The Śaiva magic tantras—spell books cataloging pragmatic rituals revealed by the god Śiva—declare that disease may be inflicted upon a victim by a malicious sorcerer; this proposition is unconsidered, perhaps rightly, by scientific epidemiology. However, the texts also declare that health, even superhuman health, can result from antidote rituals against these same diseased rites. Not all physical afflictions are caused by ill-intentioned ritual operations, but some illnesses are the result of sorcery, and, thereby, a disease that causes illness, even death, may only be the proximate cause of ill health; the ultimate cause being the hatred and jealousy of the sorcerer who performs or commissions the cruel magic ritual.[2]

After contextualizing disease in magic rituals found in Śaiva Hinduism, this chapter describes magic rituals extracted from texts in the Uḍḍ-corpus, a hybrid body whose titles all start with the syllable 'Uḍḍ-'; these texts share common lore and characteristics and are primarily concerned with aggressive magic rituals.[3] The sources are impossible to date, and while they are of a piece with medieval sources, their composition could be as late as the 19th century. Here, magic is pragmatic ritual technology. Following Mandelbaum, the pragmatic mode of religion concerns daily life, causes material changes, invokes local deities locally or translocal deities in a local manner, alters social dynamics, has a discrete result, and seeks knowledge relevant to immediate concerns; by contrast, the transcendental mode effects the soul and maintains the social structure, confers salvation, calls totranslocal deities,

DOI: 10.4324/b22930-7

often disembodied, and its rituals are performed repeatedly (1966). Compare offering a lamp to find a lost calf with performing life-cycle rituals (*saṃskāra*) or daily practices to insure the sun continues to rise (*agnihotra*). Results are brought about by rituals performed correctly, not by the power of god, the sanctity/devotion of a ritual performer, nor by supernatural power (*siddhi*) (Ullrey 2023). These rituals are a body of techniques, especially mantras, preserved in texts called tantras. Hindus often scoff at such practices, dismissing them as tantra-mantra—spellcraft quackery—and even use the English term 'black magic' in vernacular languages. At the same time, the effectiveness of these aggressive rites is widely feared.

Magic operations may inflict illness itself or deploy disease-causing entities upon victims, yet the same ritual procedures sometimes provide antidotes for hostile results. Some of these antidote rituals even bring about a supernatural state of health enabling all manner of vigor and long life, delivering powerful resistance to future disease and magical aggression. While sorcerers, filled with hatred and jealousy, deploy magic rituals, revealed by God, to harm victims, God, as seen below, also reveals simpler rituals to resolve magic affliction and disease. The knowledge of magic is understood to be essential for all humans so they might afflict others when needed, might repel magical attacks, and might become a powerful human-in-the-world. But magic is not real; at least it is not materially effective, despite the seemingly endless sources describing and prescribing it. The study of magic—more specifically, magic rituals—reveals surprising nuances to the social tensions and metaphysical suppositions of magic texts' audiences, be they practicing sorcerers, prospective clients, or authors cataloging lore. Examining magic requires imagination. Approaching any magic ritual, I first envision the ritual space and the tools deployed within it, then the different ingredients, then spells written or spoken, then actions, and I conclude by assessing how the declared effects are mirrored in each part of the operation. The most satisfying interpretations are not about magic technology but the social tensions expressed in the rites. Magic rituals' response to social tensions is usually antisocial, aggressively afflicting any who oppose the ritualist; such antisocial tendencies may be the reason magic is prohibited across cultures, the reason magic is characterized by illegality (Smith 1995).

Hinduism is hard to classify, for it has no universal scripture, comprehensive religious authority, or central doctrine; attempts to force a singular definition are mired not only in colonial presuppositions about religion but myriad encounters between those considered Hindus and those not considered Hindu (Lorenzen 1999). That said, themes and threads can be traced through Hinduisms or the Hindu traditions (Doniger 2009:17–49), and in the chapter below I examine the curious backwaters of Śaiva magic tantras.

Diseases are created by God—as all things are created by God in theistic Hinduisms—but diseases, as well, are gods (Zysk 1985:8–11). Fever and fevers, in particular, are deities and classes of deities tracing back to the earliest strata of Vedic religion (Zysk 1983). Disease-gods or demons are like hungry tigers: their nature is to attack, not out of malice but due to their very nature (Conway 1879: 7–22). Some diseases are gods, and they are not completely negative. Śitalā, the smallpox goddess, a goddess of skin eruptions, may be worshipped for general auspiciousness and luck, but one should not be too devoted, lest she come visit her disease upon the worshipper (White 2003; Stewart 1995). Diseases are conscious, non-physical entities, and those entities can be manipulated using magic.

Diseases can be cast upon victims by a sorcerer, and he—it is almost always a male acting as a sorcerer—enacts rituals to afflict, even kill, a victims. The purpose is to usurp the goods of life, long held to be the primary concern for humans: wife, children, wealth, and land. Harold Kushner asked, "Why do bad things happen to good people?" He concluded that the Jewish God is limited in power, suffering with and alongside those afflicted on earth (Kushner 1981). The magic tantras do not propose such a compassionate reading of affliction, for disease may be the result of a malicious ritual.

2 Who and What Are Diseases?

Disease in Hindu traditions challenges assumptions in Western epistemology. From the earliest South Asian medical sources, disease is considered a morbific imbalance of humors, namely an imbalance of the three humors (*doṣa*)—bile (*pitta*), wind (*vāyu*), and mucus (*śleṣman*). Humors are chemical systems in the body that influence health and well-being; they interact with the five elements: earth, air, fire, water, and space. If the three humors are balanced (*tridoṣasama*), then health occurs; otherwise, health is not established (Wujastyk 2009, xvii–xviii). Caraka argues in his pre-3rd century BCE *Compendium* (*Carakasaṃhitā*) that diseases (*roga*) are threefold: "internal," caused from the imbalanced humors; "invasive," caused by external influences and beings such as "creatures, poison, wind, fire, or wounding"; or"mental," caused by "not getting what one wants, or getting what one does not want" (Wujastyk 2009, 31). Invasive diseases are those very diseases deployed by the magic rituals in question.

Diseases are entities—dreadful entities who invade the body. Established in the physical form, they inspire symptoms. The most common invasive disease entities are the so-called seizers (*graha*); they seize an individual, visiting illness upon him or her (White 2003: 34–43; Filliozat 1963: 48–65). Included in this group are diverse creatures called fevers (*jvara*) who inflict fever (*jvara*); fever is such a paramount disease, thought to arise from the imbalance of humors, that the *Suśrutasaṃhitā* declares it 'the king of diseases' (Monier-Williams, 1872, 428). Another disease and disease demon named *takman*, found in Vedic sources (the earliest of Sanskrit scriptures), is fever and also causes fevers, especially malarial fever (Zysk 1985: 34–36).

Some diseases are divine, at least semi-divine. Magic texts abound with personified fevers (*jvara*), but these fevers are a class of dangerous entities; they are not individual gods to be worshipped. On the other hand, epilepsy (*apasmara*), the falling disease, is a divine visitation (White 2003, 1996). Other deities manifest diseases such as smallpox. Śitalā, the smallpox goddess, is considered a deity worshipped not only for relief from smallpox but to bring general prosperity (White 2003; Stewart 1995). Novel goddesses, such as the AIDS goddess, have been adopted by Hindus; older deities are associated with newly arising diseases or novel deities created outright (Dalrymple 2009, Narayanan 2000). COVID-19 deities, especially goddesses, have been reported in the press across South Asia in recent years: the Corona Mother (*coronamātā*) and the Corona Goddess (*coronadevī*).[4] Hinduisms maintain a reverence for such deities, but a devotee may not wish to revere disease deities too much, for, paradoxically, too much devotion may call that entity onto and into you: *darśana* becomes disease.

3 Sources

The text category Uḍḍ-corpus refers to inter-related texts: *Uḍḍīśatantra*, *Uḍḍāmeśvaratantra*, *Uḍḍāmareśvaratantra*, *Uḍḍāmaratantra*, and, an outlier, the *Vīrabhadratantra*. The texts' titles, in order, are translated "The Leaping Lord Tantra," "The Tantra of the Bellowing Lord,""The Tantra of the Lord who Bellows," "The Bellower Tantra," and "The Tantra of the Shining Hero." I will refer to the specific texts by their Sanskrit titles below. The prefix '*ut*' is added to the root '√*ḍī*' or '√*ḍam*' to create the '*uḍḍīś*-' or '*uḍḍām*-' syllables. Etymological similarities in titles, however, do not establish connections between Sanskrit texts; content similarities establish real connections. Much of the material below was presented in Ullrey 2016.

Uḍḍ-corpus texts reproduce not only cognate verses but identical lore. The texts share characteristic introductory verses, and similar, not identical, textual framing strategies. They share ritual content, often reproducing the same verses, but sometimes analogous rituals are presented with completely different language, i.e., they share the same lore, the common set of knowledge regarding magic rituals, but the language on the page is completely different. The Uḍḍ-corpus is incorporated by common content; all these texts are magic tantras by genre because their main contents are magic rituals. This is more than a tautology: the characteristic quality of these texts is their common contents. The weight of such similarities amounts to more than influence, more than the texts informing one another; such similarities reveal a tradition of Uḍḍ-corpus texts. These texts circulated and expanded, their content separated and combined, and they establish a South Asia-wide discourse about magic rituals.

Frequent back-and-forth borrowing prohibitively complicates any search for an Uḍḍ-corpus urtext. The literary culture producing magic tantras did not place importance on currating unique or consistent titles. I have yet to encounter a single, early source from which all, or even most, Uḍḍ-corpus texts stem. Membership in the Uḍḍ-corpus is established by sharing 'family resemblances,' not by fitting into a 'family tree' of textual development and branching recensions. These sources, not unlike medical and alchemical texts, resist placement in time and location; they lack specifics of history and geography (Goudriaan 1981: 118–120).

I will present material from four texts below, and I will refer to sources by the names of their editors; three texts have the same name, *Uḍḍīśatantra*, and are edited by Tripāṭhī (1965), Miśra (1998), and Śrivāstava (2007), respectively, and the fourth is the *Uḍḍāmareśvaratantra* edited by Zadoo, published in the Kashmir Series of Texts and Studies (1947). These are not merely three versions of the same text: the root texts are quite different, yet all of them bear common verses and ritual contents. The texts, glosses, and commentaries reveal that each source has a particular perspective guided by the editors. These four sources were published in the 20th and early 21st centuries, each drawing from notably older texts; unfortunately, none disclose those older sources or manuscripts from which these versions are edited.

4 General Statements on Disease and Magic in the *Uḍḍīśatantra*

The so-called six results (*ṣaṭkarman*), the results of aggressive magic rituals, reveal a perhaps surprising aspect of disease: disease is magically inflicted by another person, and it is often inflicted to kill. When one seeks to kill a neighbor, a disease is a useful expedient.

Yet, magic and magic rituals—those pragmatic rites that bring about aggressive results—are prohibited and illegal in Hinduism, following a pattern across cultures in which magic is illicit (Edmonds 2019: 40–52; Smith 1995: 17; Kieckhefer 1989: 176–202). Śiva declares the purpose of magic in the following verse found in both Mishra's and Srivastava's *Uḍḍīśatantra*: "Listen up, Rāvaṇa! One should practice forcible eradication (*uccāṭaṇa*) and slaying (*vadha*), by means of which home, field, wife, wealth (*dhana*), and children are seized (*hṛta*)" (Mishra 6.1, Srivastava 76). Śiva speaks about eradication and slaying, i.e., murder, but the ultimate result of eradication and slaying is the same: the victim is removed. Considering I have not located any other verses in which Śiva provides ethical regulations for aggressive magic, I argue this statement applies to all hostile magic rituals: their overall result for the sorcerer is to get rid of somebody, another rival man, and take his wealth and women.

Despite ambiguities of ethics, magic rituals and knowledge about magic rituals are essential, as Śiva states to Rāvaṇa in Tripathi's *Uḍḍīśatantra*, "Dear one, you have asked this good question for the benefit of the masses. I will reveal this tantra called the *Uḍḍīśa* in your presence." (1.2) The dangers from being afflicted by magic and the gains from deploying magic are myriad.

> When injured, what can the man do if he does not know this *Uḍḍīśa*? Should he go from where he stands up to [the peak of] mount Meru [the highest point on earth, then] the oceans will flood the earth [to reach him].
>
> (1.3)

Magic rituals make a man irrepressible, able to "fell the sun to the earth" as if using the weapons of the gods: the lightning bolt (*vajra*) of Indra, noose of Varuṇa, staff of Yama, the spear of Agni (1.4–5). Magic rituals, especially murder, should not, however, be performed lightly, for "Should a fool perform the rituals in this tantra, he will himself be assailed. Therefore, to protect oneself, nobody should perform murderous sorcery." (1.224) And, "Only a holy man (*brahmātmaṇa*), having discerned [the rituals and situation] with discriminating eyes, should ever perform murderous sorcery; otherwise, sin (*doṣa*) is incurred." (1.225) Specific rituals are classified under the term *ṣaṭkarman,* or *ṣaṭkarmāni*. The *Uḍḍāmeśvaratantra,* edited by Zadoo, argues that super-fierce methods (*mahāraudra*), including spells and occult lore, herbal manipulation, and sorcery (*abhicārika*), must be known, because they protect against wicked, injurious, vile-speaking, greedy folk from bad families (12.12–15). Should those deplorables be the only ones knowing such rituals, and, by implication, the wise are unaware of remedies, then the wicked become invincible (12.16).

Despite being called the six results, they are usually eightfold, and some texts describe a ninth result—*puṣṭi* (increasing)—that is connected to the first, *śānti* (tranquilizing). Six, eight, or eighty-eight in number, the topic is always the *ṣaṭkarman*, the 'six results.' They consist of the following:

1 *śānti-puṣṭi* (tranquilizing-increase)
2 *vaśīkaraṇa* (subjugating)
3 *stambhana* (immobilizing)
4 *mohana* (bewildering)
5 *vidveṣana* (dissent)
6 *uccāṭana* (eradicating)
7 *ākarṣaṇa* (attracting)
8 *mārana* (murder)

Explanations of each result describes variants to nuance effects; for instance, *kṣobha* (agitating) or *jñānahāni* (stupefying) are both grouped under *mohana* (bewildering). Intriguingly, disease-conferring and disease-removing techniques are often found in opening verses of any chapter on ritual results; this suggests disease was an immediate and observable aspect of magic, and its position suggests its primacy and prevalence.

Among these six results, the most important for describing disease are tranquilizing (*śānti*), murder (*mārana*), and destruction (*nāśana*). A reader may think that destruction rituals regarding disease would destroy diseases and seizers(*graha*) who cause them, yet these destructive rituals usually destroy the life and livelihood of victims, not destroying disease, and, hence, the rites are destructive in themselves. Diseases are tranquilized by *śānti* rites. Throughout the texts are found scattered remedies for magic rituals, and these return the victim to health or confer a positive state in which the target may no longer be afflicted by disease (sometimes they are immune to further magic rituals): health is being free from magic, free from disease. Below, I will explore magical health further.

Magic rituals are best studied with all the details and with rich descriptions of context interpreters ought reading complete procedures and results alongside complete procedures and results (Ullrey 2023). Prior surveys of *ṣaṭkarman* fail to adequately interpret the ritual discourse because they solely present magic ritual results without detailed procedures to enact them (Buhnemann 2000; Turstig 1985; Goudriaan 1978).

5 Specific Magic Rituals

The contents of magic tantras in this text can be categorized in two distinct ways: (1) systematic lore in which meta-ritual (ritual lore about ritual and rituals about rituals) is extracted—for instance, when different materials are described for rosary threads and beads depending on the type of ritual results desired or when the results are ranked and described in reference to one another—and (2) encyclopedic lore that presents catalogs of rituals that may be organized by the result but also may be listed without organization, sometimes categorized, sometimes just listed. By analogy, systematic lore is culinary science or gastronomy, but encyclopedic lore is recipe catalogs, like the "church cookbooks" so common in late-20th-century American congregations. Tripathi's *Uḍḍīśatantra* is divided into three parts: the first is systematic and the second is encyclopedic, and the third presents a combination of systematic and encyclopedic. Zadoo's *Uḍḍāmareśvaratantra* is mostly encyclopedic but shifts into systematic lore variously throughout the text. Other Uḍḍ-corpus texts and manuscripts contain little systematic lore, suggesting this lore is later and second order, developed to make sense out of previous lore similar to Freud's famous "secondary revision," such that initially incoherent contents are revised to create a coherent depiction. Furthermore, systematic lore initially extracted from encyclopedic catalogs could be used by authors to create innovative rituals inspired by systematic ritual principles, theoretically generating new encyclopedic rituals.

6 Systematic Lore

Disease and health lore in Tripathi's systematic section demonstrate that health is the removal of disease, for diseases are afflictive, non-corporeal creatures who have made their way into the body. States of ill health are vast, and the following verses from Tripathi explain the possible symptomatologies of a person afflicted by magic rituals.

> He is said to be immobilized, disturbed, obstructed, without power, repelled, deaf, blind, and nailed down (*kīlita*). He who is stupefied is drained, lax, fearful, filthy, reviled, split, fast asleep (*suṣupta*), and intoxicated with passion. His virility is removed; he is bereft (*hīna*). He passes despite his youth from being a child, to an adolescent, to middle

> aged, and, ultimately, he is like an old man. He is without potency and without perfection. He is lazy and fraudulent. He is poor, impure, squint-eyed (*kekara*), and his life is short. He is both obscured and devoid of qualities. He is deluded, and he hungers. He is exceptionally arrogant though devoid [of strength] in his arms. He is excessively violent. He is incredibly fierce: when his mind is at peace, he feels shame. He flees from his home, agitated; he is without affection. Such is said [about the man afflicted by the spells]. I have explained the signs of those beset by the afflictions.
>
> (2.31–37)

The result of these magic rituals is a degenerate mind, which could be extended to a state of ill mental health in modern terms, and a weak, afflicted body. The victim is not healthy. The target is afflicted.

There is a method behind the results and the rituals that confer them. Four verses at Tripathi's opening describe the symptomatology of varied results (1.10–13)—e.g., eradication (*vidveṣana*) causes mutual hatred among intimates, murder is death, and so forth. All such six-result rituals should be performed "knowing the appropriate deity, direction, and time." (1.13) Tranquilizing (*śānti*) is "the expulsion of disease (*roga*), witches (*kṛtyā*), seizers (*graha*), and so forth." (1.10) While tranquilizing removes the entities who cause disease, murder rituals "remove the life-breath of the living." (1.12) Health and life are removed. Death, the absence of health, is the supreme state of ill health. A later verse ranks the six results, though it elides tranquilizing (likely because tranquilizing was a late addition to catalogs): "murderous sorcery is greater than eradication. In fact, murderous sorcery is the greatest among all the acts. No action has ever been, nor will be, greater than murderous sorcery." (1.86–7) An altruistic ritualist might assert healing rituals are the greatest, and one modern commentator/editor argues just this (Srivastava 79–80). However, the sheer amount of murderous ritual lore and statements about the power of murder rituals suggests otherwise: murder rites are the most potent and prominent.

A wide range of magic rites to cause health or tranquilize disease use sympathetic principles by offering pleasant, tasty, appealing subjects; this contrasts aggressive magic techniques that use nasty, impure, acrid substances. Tranquilizing rites use pleasant ingredients. One tranquilizing ritual "requires a gold pot decorated with the nine jewels. If [a gold pot is] not available, a lovely pot made of copper or silver [may be used];" (1.88) and "one affects pacification after 100,000 sacrifices [of] a large amount of clarified butter, wood-apple, and sesame" (1.124).

Tranquilizing and destroying (*nāśana*) overlap; destroying is an older type of rite originally categorized under murder; but several sources re-categorize destroying under tranquilizing, and I follow them. Fever is to be destroyed (*vināśayet*) "by offerings of mango leaves;" in addition, to ward off death (*mṛtyujayana*), natural or hastened by sorcery, one should "offer *cocculus cordiflorius* (*guḍūcī*), and this also pacifies elephants and horses. Having offered white mustard, one restricts cattle disease." (1.134–5) Such ingredients are healthy and pleasant.

Rites that sympathetically confer health use ingredients considered healthy; unhealthy and noxious ingredients are used for destructive rituals. Healthy ingredients beget health; unhealthy ingredients beget ill health. Systematic lore in Tripathi establish that murder rituals use intoxicating dattura (*unmattabīja*), blood and poison, goat milk, flammable clarified butter, human flesh and bone, a victim's nail and hair trimmings; alternatively, one may oblate mustard and sesame oil, both acrid liquids. (1.127–9) Clarified butter is used in all rituals and can be considered neutral, and goat milk, also used often in erotic subjugation rituals, should not be considered beneficial like cow milk is beneficial. Negative sorcery, in general, makes offerings of prickly substances like chaff (*tuṣa*), thorns (*kaṇṭa*), cotton seeds, mustard seeds, along with salt. (1.131) Noxious and spicy, those ingredients, acrid in taste or "naturally" repulsive, are the ingredients appropriate to harm and kill.

Perhaps tranquilizing is self-explanatory to these authors, since systematic lore contains so little about *śānti*, especially regarding the context and ethics for performing tranquilizing rituals. Disease and danger, by their very nature, ought to be tranquilized, and no ethical regulations are required.

7 Encyclopedic Lore

Encyclopedic sections of magic tantras are like cookbooks. Magic recipes are set out, sometimes categorized by result; other encyclopedic catalogs have no organization, though either murder or tranquilizing are most often the first constituents; usually, when tranquilizing is first, then murder is last. I present rituals below that remedy ill health or magical affliction that I have extracted from these magical catalogs. Such rites sometimes bring about a positive state of health in addition to removing states and entities that cause suffering.

Tripathi's encyclopedic section opens with tranquilizing (*śānti*). The first mantra, recited one hundred thousand times, will surely tranquilize everything, will tranquilize all misfortune (*sarvāriṣṭa*): "Oṃ! Tranquilize! Tranquilize! Destroy all misfortune! *Svāhā*!"[5] (1.164) Tranquilizing is connected with destruction (*nāśana*), for tranquilizing destroys afflicting disease entities or even destroys rival magic. One destruction spell tranquilizes dangerous creatures (*dukṛtyāśānti*) by creating mantra-consecrated water that, when drunk, will cause the drinker to be "relieved from all disease for one year" (1.165). The mantra spell—"*Oṃ saṃsāṃsiṃsīṃsuṃsūṃsesaiṃsoṃsauṃsaṃ saḥ vaṃvāṃviṃvīṃvuṃvūṃveṃvaiṃvoṃvauṃ vaṃvaḥ haṃsaḥ amṛtavarccase svāhā*"—is made up of non-semantic seed syllables (*bīja*) and suggests a relief of digestive ailments such as diarrhea (*varcas*). Tripathi titles this ritual 'the tranquilizing of wicked creatures' (*dukṛtyāśānti*), suggesting the affliction of disease (*vyādhi*) is affliction by nasty entities requiring tranquilization.

Another seed-syllable mantra, without verbs, is classified for tranquilizing; it destroys all manner of dangerous creatures (for simplicity I will not cite the string of seeds, but I will translate the effects):

> Ghosts (*bhūta*), ghouls, wild protectors (*rakṣasa*), evil-minded men, tigers, lions, bears, jackals, snakes, elephants, horses, and all manner of beasts are destroyed by merely [repeating the spell] mentally. The power of this spell annihilates (*naśyanti*, *pralayaṃ yānti*) any and all ghosts and seizers (*bhūtavigraha*).
>
> (1.165–8).

The *Uḍḍāmareśvaratantra*, another Uḍḍ-corpus text, describes the means to compell a ghost (*bhūta*) to swiftly seize a victim. The sorcerer takes a four-finger-breadth log made of neem wood and smears it with the feces of an enemy; also, he writes the name of the victim upon that log, to which he makes offerings of smoke. The wood is burned upon a mound of charcoal (*citaṅgāra*); the ash and earth remaining is made into a figurine resembling the target; and then, on the eighth day of the dark portion of the fortnight, the sorcerer "should perform the 108 repetitions (*aṣṭottaraśata*). A ghost (*bhūta*) will swiftly seize him due to the spell (*mantreṇānena mantritaḥ*)." (1. 16–18) The spell invokes the Lord of All the Ghosts (*sarvabhūtāddhipata*), who is ugly, always furious, sharp-toothed, and accompanied by siezers (*graha*), dryads (*yakṣa*), ghosts (*bhūta*), and zombies (*betāla*) who are sent to burn, cook, and seize or cause the victim to be seized.[6] The Lord of these afflictive entities sends them, who are myriad, to incinerate the victim, and such burning actions are correlated with disease, usually fevers. This particular rite may be remedied (*pratyānaya*)—only a small percentage of magic rituals have remedies—by worshipping Śiva with clarified butter offerings and mantras, namely fumigation by the incense of bdellium (*guggula*) mixed with butter. The mantra asks Śiva to tranquilize generally (*śāntaya*) and to specifically remedy (*śamaya*) disease (*vyādhi*).[7] (1.29–30) Both the ritual and mantra are said to restore health and return the victim to health (*svāsthya*). As usual, the remedy is simpler than the ritual to create the affliction.

A subsequent ritual uses a similar method, selecting a Neem branch and writing the name of the target upon an image (*prakṛti*) using poison (*viṣa*), dattura (*unmatta*), black mustard (*rājika*), and salt (*lavaṇa*) mixed together as ink. Upon burning the image while reciting a spell dedicated to the flesh-consuming, heron-faced goddess Cāmuṇḍa, a fever ghost (*jvarabhūta*) will seize the victim.[8] (1.32–34a) However, this affliction may be removed, should the sorcerer so desire, by a simple action: "Health shall be restored by bathing the syllables of the name with milk." (1.34b–35a) A ritual immediately following causes blindness by depositing a salt consecrated with an *Uḍḍāmareśvara* mantra consecrated salt to poison food and drink.[9] (1.35b–38a)

Some rituals that bring flames—i.e., fevers—are caused by magical poisoning and may even afflict a group, even an army. Combine human skull bone and urine, head of an owl, tail of scorpion, poison (*hālāhalaka*), flesh of a white

worm, elephant and buffalo urine, and grind them, making a paste (*kalka*). This paste is consecrated with a mantra to Yama, the god presiding over death, asking him to destroy enemies.[10] Should this be placed in the food and drink of an army battalion, then all who merely touch those consumables will be burnt up, their bodies cleaved; without some form of expiation (*pratyānayanavarjita*), anyone who is so afflicted will surely die (1.57–61a). A later ritual uses a seed-syllable mantra to create fever. After repeating the mantra 10,000 times, any creature, four-footed or two-footed, is overcome by fever (*jvārādhibhūta*). Yet another seed-syllable mantra can simply consecrate water a mere 19 times, and "the victim is freed due to merely drinking, his health re-established" (12.35b–38a).

Fevers are not the only diseases that kill. "The excrement of an enemy (*ripuviṣṭa*) is put together with [excrement from a] scorpion (*vṛścika*) [in a pot] covered by a cloth and then buried. Dirt is piled on top. The enemy will die due to constipation (*malarodha*) but digging up [the pot] will return him to health." (Mishra 1.57) In a surprising turn, a ritual in the *Uḍḍāmareśvaratantra* confers baldness (*kulvīkāra*) but can also restore general health, or perhaps just return hair: "The wise one should make an image of his enemy using cow dung and ghee mixed with dust gathered from the footprint of an enemy, and even if [that enemy] is like a bull [it will be effective]." Having consecrated image with a mantra dedicated to Uḍḍāmareśvara who destroys desires, then "the victim's hair will be [as if cut] by a razor, [he will become bald.]"[11] (2.28–29b) That same spell can also be used to confer health. After covering the footprint of the enemy with sugar and ghee, the spell is repeated with offerings of cow milk, and then health shall be restored (2.30–1), which may include regrowth of hair! We men should be so lucky. A ritual, closely succeeding, causes blindness by depositing salt consecrated with an *Uḍḍāmareśvara*-mantra; that salt poisons food and drink, blinding those who consume them (2.35b–38a).[12]

Another disease conferred and remedied in the *Uḍḍāmareśvaratantra* is leprosy (*kuṣṭīkaraṇa*). Should the dark juice of the cashew extract (*bhallātaka*) plant and the *maṇḍalakārikā* plant be mixed with the blood of a house lizard (*ghṛhagoḍhā*), then "after seven days, even a vigorous man (*samedhita*) who has drunk this [tainted liquid] will become leprous." (2.38b–40) Other concoctions, of a notably more pleasant origin—the saps of the gooseberry (*dhātrī*), accacia (*khadira*), and neem (*nimba*) mixed with rock salt, honey, and ghee—may be given to the decrepit (*jīrṇa*) as a remedy. (2.41–2a) Concoctions made from common, healthy foodstuffs will make a person quite healthy (*saṃpadyate sukham*). (2.42b–43) Another ritual takes up an aquatic creature (*jalajīva*) and ritually dries it out; it is used to make a victim feel burning heat-pain (*atape*), as if burned by the sun, but he may be revived by bathing his body with sour rice gruel (*kāñjika*), clear water, or sesame oil gathered as remaining from the worship of a *liṅga*, the non-anthropomorphic form of Śiva as a phallus (2.43–47a).

One complicated final ritual that revivifies the dead (*saṃjīvana*) is presented at the end of Tripathi's *Uḍḍīśatantra*; rites to return the living from

the dead are often presented at the end of ritual catalogs. This ritual is particularly suited to death caused by disease, snakes, and so forth. The *aghora* mantra, or the pleasant spell, is perfected by 100,000 repetitions while seated in a cremation ground. "Oṃ! [Reverence] to the beautiful ones, the terrifying ones, to those more terrible than the terrifying! Reverences to them all! Reverence to all the arrow-throwing ones!" A summary of the ritual is found below. Operating under an *amkola* tree [bot. *Alangium hexapetalum*], after perfecting the mantra, the sorcerer worships a *liṅga*, and an unfired pot (*nava ghaṭa*), and then he winds a single thread (*sutra*) around the tree, the *liṅga*, and the pot. Four practitioners prostrate and worship using the perfected *mantra*; then, ripened fruits and flowers are gathered, cooked, and used to fill the pot. The pot is worshipped with offerings of sandal (*gaṃdha*), flowers, and unbroken grains. Having removed the chaff (*tuṣa*) from the seeds (*bīja*), he applies them to the jar's mouth that is then covered with a large plate (*bṛhaṇaṃ vṛttaṃ*); the plate smeared with auspicious substances and dirt gathered from a potter's hand (*kumbhakārakara*). Seed garlands are strung atop the pot. When dry, a copper pot is put on top and another underneath. Cook this in hot oil (*taila*) and save the oil. A half portion of that oil is combined with an equal part sesame oil (*tilatailaka*). After cooling, the oil is applied to a corpse, and the corpse will immediately return to life or go favorably to the land of Yama. Those killed by snakes (*sarpa*), disease (*roga*), and the like, they will surely return to life. (2.99–107)

8 Concluding Remarks: Who Hates You?

Uncomfortable conclusions arise from imagining these rituals. The Uḍḍ-corpus argues, as established above, that magic is to be undertaken out of hatred and jealousy; the sorcerer or his client performs the magic operation that he may usurp family and wealth of a victim. While the proximate cause of a victim's symptomatology may be a disease, the ultimate cause may be the hatred of the sorcerer.

An insightful comparison is found among the Azande people, documented in Evans-Pritchard's classic ethnography *Witchcraft, Oracles, and Magic among the Azande*. When a person is afflicted by witchcraft, signified by an unnatural or particularly persistent illness or set of bad events, a diviner will ask his client, "Who hates you?" (Evans-Pritchard 1976: 46–48) The deep cause of a weird, malicious state, including an uncanny illness, is witchcraft, and witchcraft is ultimately caused by hatred and jealousy. In a classic example, it is not odd that a grain tower falls over, but it is odd that a structure falls over at the exact moment a person is resting below that structure: that a person is struck by the falling siloh suggests witchcraft (ibid. 22). Should a spear strike a person, the spear striking is the cause of death, but the 'second spear,' the reason the spear struck at all, is witchcraft (ibid. 25–28). It is not out of the ordinary to contract a disease, but perhaps to contract a novel disease, such as COVID-19, at a very specific time suggests witchcraft,

and witchcraft is deployed out of hate and jealousy. Magic rituals causing diseases, in the same way, are performed by the hateful and jealous sorcerer who seeks to usurp the place of those laid low by his craft. Diseases are ever-existing, circulating as non-corporeal entities in search of a person to afflict, but not due to their own hatred, for disease entities are not intentional; diseases afflict due to their nature. Tigers stalk, fish swim, and, likewise, disease creatures cause illness.

If we follow the curious logic of the Uḍḍ-corpus, COVID-19 was created by God: all things, beneficent or malicious, are created by God. But the reason for COVID-19 afflicting a specific person, it could be argued, is the hatred of a sorcerer, though this hardly explains massive infections spreading across the population. As COVID-19 spread wildly, some could argue, perhaps its lethality was influenced by magic rituals upon a group or region. Or, perhaps, this COVID-19 disease emerged and spread to the world because some arch-sorcerer wished to afflict all humanities. COVID deities and COVID removing rituals are reported throughout the news, so it would not be surprising that sorcerers are suspected to secretly craft COVID-19 inflicting spells, and those sorcerers deploying spells would do so based on long-standing ritual lore to impart disease, especially fevers, as found in the Uḍḍ-corpus. I have not encountered such rites in contemporary magic tantras, and I doubt they will appear in print, though I would not be surprised to find an entrepreneurial sorcerer advertising such sources via the internet and social media.

This is an unpleasant position, but it is consistent with these tantras. Disease-granting rituals are revealed by God for the purpose of harming unwitting victims; they are to be deployed by hateful and jealous, even petty, sorcerers. But the Uḍḍ-corpus is not as pessimistic as this argument suggests. Scattered throughout the tantras are antidotes to hostile rituals. Those antidote techniques are often simpler ritual exertions using pleasant substances, contrasting the complicated rites with nasty ingredients. Those antidotes sometimes do more than just remove an affliction conferred by the sorcerer; they confer states of superhuman vigor and imperviousness to future disease. While Śiva, on the one hand, reveals an incredible variety of intricate rituals for the petty sorcerer, he also, on the other hand, provides simple counteractions that thwart aggressive magic. It seems easier to heal than to kill. It bears repeating that Tripathi's Uḍḍīśatantra declares,

> When injured, what can the man do if he does not know this Uḍḍīśa? Should he go from where he stands up to [the peak of] mount Meru [the highest point on earth, then] the oceans will flood the earth [to reach him].
>
> (1.3)

While the Uḍḍ-corpus sets out every means to magically manipulate and harass the social world, it also provides, elusively, all the means to stop the sorcerer and gain freedom from affliction.

Notes

1 I use the term Hinduisms, in plural, to note that Hinduism is not a monolithic category or even a particularly good umbrella term for the many practices performed by those who worship Hindu gods.
2 The term operation refers to the full range of a magic ritual. The operator (sorcerer) performs actions including preparing a space, setting out ingredients, rendering and speaking verbal or written spells.
3 See Ullrey (2023) for a more extensive treatment of magic rituals not limited to those related to disease.
4 Srinivas, Tulasi. "India's Goddesses of Contagion Provide Protection in the Pandemic – Just Don't Make Them Angry." "Corona Mata and the Pandemic Goddesses." "'Corona Devi': Indian Priests Pray for Mercy from Covid 'Goddess'."
5 Mantra: *oṃ śānte śānte sarvāriṣṭanāśini svāhā*
6 Mantra: *Oṃ namo bhagavate sarvabhūtādhipataye virūpākṣāya nityaṃ krūrāya daṃṣṭriṇe vikarāline grahayakṣabhūtabetālena saha śaṅkara manuṣya dahadaha pacapaca gṛhṇagṛhṇa gṛhṇāpayagṛhṇāpaya huṃ phaṭ svāhā*
7 Mantra: *Oṃ namaḥ śivāya śāntāya prabhāya muktāya devādhidevāya śubhrabāhave vyādhiṃ śamayaśamaya amukaḥ svatho bhavatu namo'stu te* (1.30)
8 Mantra: *Oṃ bakāmukhā cāmuṇḍa amukasya kṣīramāṃsaśoṇitabhojanī amukaṃ svaḥ svaḥ jvareṇa grhṇagrhṇa gṛhṇāpaya gṛhṇāpaya huṃ phaṭ svāhā*
9 Mantra: *Oṃ nama uḍḍāmareśvarāya śarīraṃ andhaṃ kuru ṭhaḥ ṭhaḥ svāhā*
10 Mantra: *Oṃ hrīṃ yamāya śatrunāśanāya svāhā*
11 Mantra: *Oṃ namo bhagavate uḍḍāmareśvarāya kāmaprabhañjanāya amuka cchaḥ cchaḥ svāhā*
12 Mantra: *Oṃ nama uḍḍāmareśvarāya śarīraṃ andhaṃ kuru ṭhaḥ ṭhaḥ svāhā*

Bibliography

Buhnemann, Gudrun, "The Six Rites of Magic," in *Tantra in Practice*, edited by David Gordon White, Princeton, NJ: Princeton University Press, 2000, 447–462.

Conway, Moncure Daniel, *Demonology and Devil-Lore*, London: Chatto and Windus, 1879.

"'Corona Devi': Indian Priests Pray for Mercy from Covid 'Goddess'," Coronavirus Pandemic News | Al Jazeera, Al Jazeera, May 27, 2021. https://www.aljazeera.com/news/2021/5/27/corona-devi-indian-priests-pray-for-mercy-from-covid-goddess.

"Corona Mata and the Pandemic Goddesses," The Wire, n.d. https://thewire.in/culture/corona-mata-and-the-pandemic-goddesses. https://theconversation.com/indias-goddesses-of-contagion-provide-protection-in-the-pandemic-just-dont-make-them-angry-139745

Dalrymple, William, *Nine Lives : In Search of the Sacred in Modern India*, London: Bloomsbury, 2009.

Doniger, Wendy, *The Hindus: An Alternative History*, New York: Penguin Press, 2009.

Edmonds III, Radcliffe G., *Drawing Down the Moon*, Princeton, NJ: Princeton University Press, 2019.

Evans-Pritchard, E.E., *Witchcraft, Oracles, and Magic Among the Azande*, Oxford: Oxford University Press, 1976.

Filliozat, Jean, *Etude De Démonologie Indienne : Le Kumāratantra De Rāvana Et Les Textes Parallèles Indiens Tibétains Chinois Cambodgien Et Arabe*, Impr. Nationale, 1937.

Goudriaan, Teun, *Māyā Divine and Human*, Delhi: Motilal Banarsidas, 1978.
Goudriaan, Teun, and Sanjukta Gupta, *Hindu Tantric and Śākta Literature*, Wiesbaden: Harrassowitz, 1981.
Kieckhefer, Richard, *Magic in the Middle Ages*, Cambridge: Cambridge University Press, 1989.
Kushner, Harold S., *When Bad Things Happen to Good People*, New York: Avon, 1981.
Lorenzen, David N., "Who Invented Hinduism?" *Comparative Studies in Society and History*, vol. 41, no. 4, 1999, 630–659.
Mandelbaum, David G., "Transcendental and Pragmatic Aspects of Religion," *American Anthropologist*, vol. 68, no. 5, 1966, 1174–1191.
Miśra, Śivadatta, *Uḍḍiśatantram: "Śivadattī"Hindīvyākhyāvibhūṣitam*, Vārāṇasī: Kṛṣṇadāsa Akādamī, 1998.
Monier-Williams, Monier, *A Sanskṛit-English Dictionary Etymologically and Philologically Arranged with Special Reference to Greek Latin Gothic German Anglo-Saxon and Other Cognate Indo-European Languages*, Oxford: Clarendon Press, 1872.
Narayanan, Vasudha, "Diglossic Hinduism: Liberation and Lentils," *Journal of the American Academy of Religion* 68, no. 4, 2000, 761–779.
Smith, Jonathan Z., "Trading Places," in *Ancient Magic and Ritual Power*, edited by Marvin Meyer and Paul Mirecki, Leiden: Brill, 1995, 11–27.
Stewart, Tony K., "Encountering the Smallpox Goddess: The Auspicious Song of Śitalā," *Religions of India in Practice*, Princeton, NJ: Princeton University Press, 1995, 389–398.
Srinivas, Tulasi, "India's Goddesses of Contagion Provide Protection in the Pandemic – Just Don't Make Them Angry," *The Conversation*, September 13, 2022.
Śrivāstava, C.M., *Uḍḍīśa* Taṃtra Sādhana Evaṃ Prayog, New Delhi: Manoj Publications, 2007.
Tripāṭhī, Śyāmasundaralāla, *Uḍḍīśatantra*, Mahārāṣṭra: Gangāviṣṇu Śrīkṛṣṇadāsa, 1965.
Turstig, Hans-Georg, "The Indian Sorcery Called Abhicāra," *Wiener Zeitschrift für die Kunde Südasiens für Indische Philosophie* 29, 1985, 69–117.
Ullrey, Aaron Michael, "Grim Grimoires: Pragmatic Ritual in the Magic Tantras," PhD diss., University of California Santa Barbara, 2016.
Ullrey, Aaron Michael, "Magic Rituals," *Brill's Encyclopedia of Hinduism*, edited by Knut Jacobsen, Leiden: Brill, 2023.
White, David Gordon, *Kiss of the Yoginī*, Chicago, IL: University of Chicago Press, 2003.
Wujastyk, Dominik, *The Roots of Ayurveda:Selections from Sanskrit Medical Writings*, Rev. ed., London: Penguin Books, 2009.
Zadoo, Jagaddhar, *Uḍḍāmareśvaratantra* (KSTS), Srinagar: Normal Press, 1947.
Zysk, Kenneth G., "Fever in Vedic India," *Journal of the American Oriental Society*, vol. 103, no. 3, 1983, 617–621.
Zysk, Kenneth G., "Religious Healing in the Veda," *Transactions of the American Philosophical Society*, vol. 75, no. 7, 1985, i–xv, xvii, 1–311.

6 "Can a Virus Destroy the Sacred?" The Latvian Experience of Holy Communion during COVID-19

Ilze Ūdre, Dace Balode and Linards Rozentāls

1 Introduction

The year 2020 brought sudden changes in the way that the modern world works, and these changes affected Lutheran parishes in Latvia, too, including their social life and their church services.

Ritual and practice have always been some of the most meaningful ways of passing on the Christian faith. Even though foundational texts and their unwritten interpretations are important means of conveying the truth, rituals also do it for those who practice them. Participation in a ritual often becomes the most significant part of one's experience, giving the most intense feeling of God's presence; it becomes the essential defining factor for one's identity.

This article is based on a survey of parish officials done by Ilze Ūdre and on the experiences of the authors in their own parishes. We were interested in specific experiences. Our guiding questions were: how do rituals change through the actual experience? Are there limits to changes in rituals, and at what point would Holy Communion lose something essential due to such changes? After we discuss the material and the methods we have used, we present some of the dilemmas. In the introduction, the characteristics of Latvian Lutherans are briefly outlined (3). The main part of our report consists of a study focused on the practice of Holy Communion in the Latvian Evangelical Lutheran Church during the pandemic. In order to discover the changes, attention will first be paid to Holy Communion Theology and Practice in the ELCL before COVID-19 (4). It will be briefly revealed how the established restrictions affected the opportunities to gather and celebrate Holy Communion in 2020–2021 (5) and what impact it had on accessibility and location (6) and type and time (7) and how it was evaluated by representatives of the churches (8).

This study, which is based on interviews conducted with representatives of ELCL congregations, is complemented by two in-depth analyses in which the practice is observed throughout the restrictions: Example No. 1: Riga Luther Evangelical Lutheran Parish (ELCL) (9) and Example No. 2: Riga Evangelical Parish Evangelical Lutheran Church Worldwide (LELCW) (10). These in-depth views allow us to get closer to the examples of digitization in

DOI: 10.4324/b22930-8

Latvian Lutheran practice. Finally, we end this study with conclusions about Holy Communion practice in Latvian Lutheran congregations (11).

2 Method and Material

To explain our perspective, a short note on our scholarly identity: we, the authors, also belong to the Lutheran tradition and come from different Lutheran churches in Latvia ELCL and LELCW.

In May 2021, a qualitative survey was conducted in the Faculty of Theology at the University of Latvia. Ilze Ūdre, while developing her bachelor's thesis, "Holy Communion practice of ELCL during the COVID-19 pandemic" (thesis defended on June 7, 2021), conducted a survey with the objective to record Holy Communion practices that were adopted during COVID-19 in the parishes of the Latvian Lutheran church. This study used 110 phone semi structured interviews with parish leaders, i.e., representatives of 38% of the registered parishes of ELCL. The method of the interviews was chosen to increase the number of interview participants. The interviews were conducted in parishes of cities, towns, and villages from all geographical regions of Latvia, and the information was evaluated in relation to the total membership number as it appears in the statistics of the Lutheran church. The survey also recorded what the people receiving the communion thought of these changes in the distribution, i.e., whether the changes in the format of Holy Communion likewise changed other aspects. The interviews lasted between 7 and 25 minutes; they were transcribed, and anonymized material was provided to the co-researchers for further analysis for the current study.

Until the beginning of the COVID-19 pandemic, four of the 110 surveyed parishes had more than 100 people attending services, 13 parishes had 50–100 people in regular attendance, 12 parishes had 21–30 people, 48 parishes had 9–20 people, and 15 had 1–8 people.

From those who regularly attended service, Holy Communion was received by more than 100 people in three parishes; in seven parishes, it was 50–100 people; in 16 parishes 31–50 people, 15 parishes 21–30 people, in 49 parishes 9–20 people received the communion, but in 20 parishes it was 1–8 people. These data show the overall situation in the Lutheran parishes in Latvia: the aging of the population and the emptying of the smaller settlements. Due to aging of the parishioners, until the beginning of the pandemic, almost 20% parishes had less than 10 people gathering together regularly.

In order to deepen the view of the practice of the Lord's Supper, two in-depth studies have also been carried out in two Lutheran congregations in which we are involved ourselves. For observation, we raised the following questions – how has practice changed, whether and how digital solutions are used, and what would be the theological implications for the future?

Both methodological approaches, interviews and observation, should help to answer the main question of our study: how the churches handled the new situation, in particular in relation to the Holy Communion.

3 Touching the Holy: Latvian Evangelical Lutheran Church and Holy Communion

A variety of different Lutheran churches exist in the country of Latvia. They do not, however, have a unified ecclesiological structure or eucharistic theology, and with regard to the latter, one would have to take into account different historical developments in a particular Lutheran church. Even within one Lutheran tradition, there could be different understandings and practices of Holy Communion. Furthermore, Lutheranism today is affected by scholarly research, but the actual practice is informed by other factors as well, including ecumenical dialogue.[1]

Looking at the ELCL in the context of other churches, one can observe that historically it has been influenced by German Lutheranism, but in the question of the Eucharist it resembles more the Swedish Church: the Eucharist can be consecrated only by an ordained pastor, and it is important for the ordination to maintain apostolic succession. Moreover, the Eucharistic elements are handled with great reverence even after the service, a practice that comes from the understanding of real presence in Holy Communion.[2]

To understand the position of the Latvian Lutheran church on the theology and practice of the Eucharist, we should take into consideration that, starting from 1940, Latvia was an occupied country and was part of the USSR. At the end of the 1980s and the beginning of the 1990s, "the Church had to define its identity anew. The Soviet occupation regime that had lasted for 46 years had mostly destroyed those traditions of ELCL and the Lutheranism that had been at the pre-war Latvia."[3] We also have to take into account that Lutheran theology in Latvia continued in a sort of ghetto state; the European theological discourses did not reach it for the most part. In this survival regime, theology just like the practice of the church was focused on survival.[4] This conservative character still marks the ELCL nowadays.

The Second World War and the occupation forced many members of the Latvian Lutheran church into exile. Around 55% of Latvian pastors were forced to leave their country.[5] The church continued its work abroad and formed the Latvian Evangelical Lutheran Church (LELC) outside Latvia. In 2016, this church established its chapter in Latvia as well. Thus, nowadays, there are both branches of the former pre-war LELC present in Latvia: ELCL and LELCW. Our research and our interest are mostly about the Eucharistic practices in the ELCL; the survey discussed below was also done in its parishes. The LELCW is represented in a further section of this article that offers a detailed analysis of an example from one of its parishes in Latvia.

4 Holy Communion Theology and Practice in the ELCL before COVID-19

One of the best sources for the current Eucharistic theology and practice of the ELCL is its council's regulations on celebrating Holy Communion, published in 1998.[6] These regulations determine in detail the liturgical tools used at Holy Communion (dishes and textiles), how to prepare the elements, their consecration and distribution, and the reception of different communions. For example, the regulations say that the communicant should receive the Eucharist on his or her knees, they explain in detail what to do with the leftovers (the consecrated cannot be mixed with the un-consecrated, it may not be discarded into an ordinary rubbish, there are special regulations what to do if the wine has a foreign substance in it). It also regulates that a pastor has the authority to exclude a parish member from the Eucharistic communion if the person in question "lives in open sin." In general, these regulations come from a strong understanding of substantial real presence in the elements that lasts after the end of the service, and they are meant to ensure the sacred nature and protection of the Eucharist. These regulations do not talk about the horizontal aspect of the Eucharist, namely the formation of the communion among the communicants. However, the regulations affirm that the elements of the Eucharist should be received by all communicants together, using one single cup.

Theological positions were established at several pastoral conferences before the regulations were accepted where the questions regarding the Eucharist were discussed. They show a certain attitude about the frequency of celebrating the Eucharist: ELCL pastors defend a position that it should not be consumed only once a year but as often as the faithful would like. The discussions show that the pastors held a general understanding of the substantial divine real presence in the elements. Some pastors defended the view that the presence of Christ in the Eucharistic elements remains until their complete annihilation, whereas there were also pastors who believed that the special presence of Christ ceases at the end of the Eucharist.[7]

In the context of COVID-19, it is interesting to see that at the end of 1990s, there was a discussion by the pastors on whether to use one or several cups. It was pointed out that, because of hygiene reasons, the use of one cup might be problematic.[8] There was a suggestion that this could be solved by using the intinction method, i.e., dipping bread into wine, a practice widely used in the East. The participants of the discussion rejected it on the grounds that such a practice would differ from the description of the Last Supper in the Gospels. In these Lutheran discussions, there is a reference to a Catholic doctrinal element as well: this practice apparently lacks the element of sacrifice, i.e., "blood is not separated from the body."[9]

The discussion is not followed by specific conclusions; the argument in favor of different cups was made in response to hygiene concerns, but the argument for one cup was based on the example of Jesus. Separate cups were seen as destroying the symbol of unity and considered an innovation, which was against the traditional Lutheran loyalty to church traditions.[10]

Despite these discussions that are interesting to read in the light of modern concerns regarding COVID-19, the interviews conducted for this research showed that the church regulations published in 1998 were regarded as general recommendations; for our current context, this meant that parishes before and after the pandemic were free to adjust them to their own needs and their own understanding of the Eucharist.

5 Can a Virus Destroy the Sacred? Changes during COVID-19 in Latvian Lutheran Churches

COVID-19 grew into a global pandemic within five months. It made governments worldwide to react rapidly to this new threat to their societies. There was no precedent of decisions being made so fast and of such a scale in the modern world. These decisions affected individuals and communities, including churches.[11] When COVID-19 reached Latvia, the Lutheran church initially encouraged to practice only minimal caution in the church. After the state of emergency in Latvia was declared, the ELCL also reacted, ruling that until Easter of 2020 all church services should be canceled. This ruling marked the beginning of the first COVID-19 wave in the Latvian Lutheran parishes.

On March 17, 2020, only a few days after the emergency state was declared, an almost comical agreement was achieved between the state and the church: services with a very small number of people were allowed but could not be advertised. Information about religious services were taken down from all channels of information; new formulations appeared, such as "the pastor serves at the usual time." It meant that, at the usual church service time that regular parish members were familiar with from pre-COVID-19 days, the pastor would lead a service in the church. It could be attended by a small number of people, only up to the number allowed in the building. Many parishes continued this practice throughout the pandemic, insisting that a church service is not a public event but for an exclusive group of people, the parish. Several Lutheran pastors criticized this approach as this interpretation of the ban on public events was against the essence of the ban: to restrict the gathering and movement of people.

May 12, 2020, can be regarded as the end of the first COVID-19 wave in Latvia when the government lifted the state of emergency. Even though not all restrictions on indoor and outdoor gatherings were lifted, a larger number of people were allowed to congregate. Regulations on the particulars of gathering were changed several times during the summer of 2020, allowing church services outdoors and increasing the number of people who could be in a church building. However, in autumn 2020, when the numbers of those infected by COVID-19 grew, government institutions reinstated restrictions on the number of people in churches and issued an order for mandatory usage of face masks.

During the second wave of the pandemic from November 2020 until March 2021, church services were not canceled officially, but they were not advertised. Therefore, they were attended by a comparatively small number of people. If services did take place, they typically included Holy Communion.

6 Change in the Practice of Holy Communion in 2020–2021: Accessibility and Location

The survey shows that, during the first COVID-19 wave, the situation of Latvian Lutheran parishes changed considerably. At this time, about half of the surveyed parishes canceled their services for up to 12 weeks. It was impossible, therefore, to receive the communion; likewise, all the other activities in churches were canceled, including Alfa courses, confirmation courses, prayer meetings, etc. Parish chairpersons explained that, during the first COVID-19 wave in particular, there was lots of confusion and uncertainty in the society.

> People were busy with their own concerns. The communication in the parish continued, of course, we organized prayer groups that used WhatsApp, the pastor was sending out words of encouragement. At that time prayers substituted everything else that we used to do as a parish,[12]

remembers one of the parish leaders reflecting on the beginning of COVID-19.

During the first COVID-19 wave, 36 parishes of those surveyed did not offer communion. The following reasons were cited: worship services were not taking place, the pastor did not live near the parish, or there were no clear directives from church authorities on how to take the communion under these circumstances. None of the participants called this abstention from the Eucharist "fasting from the Eucharist" due to the pandemic restrictions. We had greater concerns than to worry about receiving the communion. The main thing was and still is the small number of people [in the parish]. The main thing was to keep people together, so that there would be a parish, remembers a parish leader from a small town.

The majority of the respondents were employing different ways of receiving Holy Communion during the pandemic. In 39 parishes, the communion could be received individually. There were several forms for this individual Eucharist. In some parishes, it was distributed when the pastor stayed in the church for some hours after a service that was broadcast online. That way, the communion could be received individually in the parishes where services were canceled. "People did not give up the communion because of COVID. Of course, numbers went down, but people still used the opportunity to go to the church on Sundays to see the pastor and receive the communion at certain hours," explained a leader of a city parish. However, in smaller towns and villages, the situation was different. There was a very small number of people who used the opportunity to receive Holy Communion individually.

Several pastors remember this period of individual Eucharist as very intensive and peculiar. A pastor of one town told that it was like having a Eucharistic service with each person and each family separately. They read the gospel, recited together the words of the Eucharistic prayer, and said the Lord's prayer as well as the prayer of confession. "When there are 30–40 people at the communion, it is not possible to be so close together with each one, but during the COVID it was more unique," one of the pastors remembered his work.

The respondents did not hide that in order to adjust to the new situation they needed some initiative, skills, and also funds, particularly with regard to digital solutions for the services, prayer meetings, and access to the digital Eucharist. Therefore, it was particularly difficult for the parishes that had a smaller number of regular participants in the services even before the pandemic to adapt to the COVID-19 situation, as it meant they had less funds to install the equipment to help during the pandemic. These parishes also had a greater number of elderly parish members (meaning less skills and will to use digital devices), and they did not have their own pastor who would offer solutions and inspire the parishioners to be more active in adjusting to the new situation. The usage of digital devices during the first COVID-19 wave marked the division between those who attended services regularly and received Holy Communion versus those who did not. During the first COVID-19 wave in the parishes that broadcast their services, it was noticeable that there was less participation from seniors. During summer 2020, another trend was noticeable. During worship services, some members of the congregation were in the church while some were at home on their digital devices; yet, both groups participated in the same service. Several parish chairpersons explained that, in most cases, it was the Eucharist that made people attend services in person.

> For those who watch services on Facebook or parish website, there was no option offered to come at a different time to receive the communion. The people who wanted to receive the communion came to the service where at the end we all received it,

explained a parish chairperson from one town. In another city parish, an option was offered to receive the communion after the service for those people who participated in this service remotely. However, there was very little interest in this option, and the parish chairperson concluded that those people who wanted communion participated in the service in person.

In summer 2020, when the spread of the virus diminished and the national state of emergency was canceled, only eight parishes did not return to services in person. These were small parishes on the countryside with high numbers of elderly people and also the parishes where the first COVID-19 wave had affected so many people that it was agreed with the pastors not to renew regular services in person. A total of 102 of the surveyed parishes resumed services in person; 19 of these parishes also continued to broadcast their services.

7 Changes in the Practice of Holy Communion in 2020–2021: Type and Time

COVID-19 affected Eucharist practice with regard to its distribution, how people received it, and the way individual absolution was done without the pastor touching the communicants.[13] Because of the pandemic, in parishes where the Eucharist was distributed during the service, the communicants went to the altar individually, with other family members, or in small groups. During the first wave of COVID-19, pastors disinfected their hands after each communicant. During the second wave, many pastors distributed the Eucharist wearing a face mask, but the communicants took off their masks only briefly while receiving the communion. During the surveyed period, there was no physical contact between the communicant and the pastor in any of the parishes.

At the beginning of COVID-19, the council of the Latvian Lutheran church suggested that congregations distribute the communion by intinction.[14] Most of the parishes, particularly those outside the bigger cities, followed this advice, if not at the beginning, then later in the pandemic, when they switched from their traditional practices to those suggested by the ELCL. In the parishes where it was decided to follow other practices, in most cases the decisions about how to act were made by pastors and parishes discussing them together, i.e., the parishes themselves had an opportunity to express their opinion about their individual preferences.

Among all the parishes that were surveyed in spring 2021, the Eucharist was received by intinction in 99 of them; 11 parishes had a different practice. Seven parishes in smaller Latvian towns and settlements did not use the intinction, opting instead for another type of distribution.[15] One of these parishes used individual cups for the distribution of the consecrated wine; the words of the consecration were spoken while the wine was in a communal cup, and then it was poured into the smaller cups. Another practice was to use spoons. Several parishes used individual cups at the beginning of the pandemic but considered it inconvenient for different reasons and switched to intinction later.

In a small town, the pastor met with every communicant (either individual or a family) and read the gospel; together, they spoke the words of consecration and said the Lord's prayer and the prayer of confession. The pastor decided to do so after asking himself: what can I do to respond to people's needs?

> From the phone calls and conversations, it could be felt that the presence of the pandemic is existential in people's lives. All conversations were very deep, everything was on a completely new level. Those were

> conversation about the essential meanings: is this the end of the world, is this God's will? Suddenly there was a real understanding in people's lives about Christ's presence. Especially at the beginning of the pandemic there was a real feeling of meaning of faith and trust,

told the parish pastor. In summer 2020, when it was possible for the parishioners to meet again, the members of this congregation received the Eucharist from a communal cup as it was before the pandemic. However, at the beginning of the second wave of COVID-19, the pastor introduced intinction.

A parish in Riga with a much larger congregation decided that intinction was not a good solution. Since the beginning of the COVID-19 pandemic, this parish had discontinued Holy Communion during the in-person services, only to offer it separately. Participants received the communion individually; therefore, the communal cup was used in the same way as before COVID-19. The only difference was that the Eucharist was not received by the entire congregation together but individually; in addition, the cup was disinfected after each recipient had been served.

In the surveyed parishes that were close to the median size of the ELCL parishes in general, a possibility of a digital form of the Eucharist had not been actively discussed. During the time of the survey, only one parish distributed the Eucharist by means of technologies. That reflects the particular situation in Latvia: parishes are not large, and they are local. Even the parishes in towns are easily accessible in terms of distance. Hence, for most Latvian parishes, Holy Communion was an important in-person event even in the time of crisis because, as the respondents explained, the congregation came together in person precisely for the reason of communion.

8 "It's Good That Holy Communion and Services Are Happening At All": The View of Parish Officials About the Differences in the Practice of Holy Communion

According to the information gathered during the interviews, some parishioners had been involved in discussions on the organization of the Eucharist, whereas elsewhere, everything was decided by the pastor alone. In addition, most of the respondents stated that the meaning of the sacrament remained the same regardless of a changing practice (89 from 110 responses). However, parish officials in five parishes emphasized that the Eucharist has lost some of its importance because of COVID-19 restrictions.

One of the main changes in their experience of communion pertained to the usage of the common cup, as is the tradition in the Latvian Lutheran church. According to one of the parish leaders in the interview,

> Those who have the need for the sacrament accept the circumstances the way they are. Everybody understands the circumstances. It is not the case that people would not take the communion because there is no

> cup, but one is left with the feeling that it is not a fully valid sacrament because there is no communal cup. It was not as satisfying as the way it used to be when the sacrament was used by everybody together.

Several other parish leaders also emphasized that the communal cup was the essence of the sacrament and that the Eucharist was important for the community: "It is good that the Eucharist and services happen at all. However, the new practice has of course changed something; there is not the sort of community feel as it was before the pandemic." Another parish leader was critical about the intinction. According to her, intinction "crippled" the sacrament. "It is a physical feeling when you receive the body and blood of Christ, you feel that it is inside you. But in the intinction you receive body and blood together. It is a completely different physical feeling," she stated, not hiding her opinion.

In other interviews, however, people expressed the opinion that an individually received Holy Communion is even more meaningful. A parish leader from a small town said that, in his opinion, Holy Communion received individually is more meaningful than the one received together with others:

> Holy Communion is the most solemn moment in the whole service and now I can go by myself and receive it. For me it is more uplifting, more solemn than to go to the communion with others. I think that COVID forced us to find new ways how to approach God. Because even new practice is a way to approach God in all times and in different circumstances.

A chairperson of one parish explained that, in many countries, Christians suffer because church services due to COVID-19 are canceled completely. It is important that in Latvia they could take place and people could receive communion. Even though many respondents mentioned the lack of a common Eucharist and the common cup as a drawback, the general feeling was well described by one respondent:

> It is very hard to inspire people to a fellowship if there are so many riches in the worldly life. At the same time, especially in the COVID-19 situation, worship, sacrament, and being in the church are really necessary in order to resist, to unite 'here and now' with that which is above the worldly life,

meaning to revisit one's life's priorities, strengthen one's faith against the challenges that one has to meet daily.

Most of the respondents said that parishioners considered the year of the pandemic as only a temporary solution to a crisis; changes were not viewed to be permanent. "A Lutheran receives what he (*sic*) receives. Even when he does not receive the sacrament the usual way. Faith is the root of every sacrament therefore intinction as a solution for a crisis situation is acceptable," a parish chairperson explained his position. Somebody else added: "The essence of the Holy Sacrament is that you receive Christ's body and blood. The essence is in the reception not in the way you receive it." Another parish leader pointed out that if it was only eating and drinking, then we could talk about changes, but at Holy Communion one unites with Jesus, not bread and wine. Therefore, changes in the practice do not change anything. "The Sacrament has not lost its value because this mess caused by people or allowed by God cannot change the essence of the Eucharist. There is a presence of the Spirit there and nobody has any doubts about it." Similarly, "Nowhere in the Bible does it say how much wine one should be drinking to know that there has been enough. Even if there is only one drop, there is no difference. It is rather a question of tradition, the usage of the common cup, it is symbolic, and it shows that we are all in Christ, that the Church is the body of Christ. There should be bread and wine in the communion, and it does not matter how much."

The survey shows that most congregations accepted changes in the practice so that they could receive communion at all and while it was offered in both kinds, they did not see any difference. However, during the research the congregations did not consider the practices during COVID-19 as permanent. In many conversations, people expressed the hope that they could return to the common cup and the previous, familiar Eucharistic practices. Statistically, a very small number of respondents acknowledged that the new solutions could be permanent because of different reasons: hygiene or spread of infection in the future, and also because it could be a barrier for younger people to join the church for reasons of comfort and safety over some centuries-old traditions.

The COVID-19 pandemic showed an interesting nuance with regard to space. Because of country-wide regulations, large and small parishes found themselves at equal footing because gatherings were not regulated by the size of the parish but rather by floor space and allowed people to come together depending on how much distance they could keep. In terms of continuing their practices in person, smaller parishes had an advantage. However, thinking about how this time had influenced the size of parishes and their future developments, one has to conclude that bigger and technologically more advanced parishes could increase in size by COVID-19 as they could reach out to people using digital media.

9 In-Depth Analysis Example No. 1: Riga Luther Evangelical Lutheran Parish (ELCL)

When during the first COVID-19 pandemic wave inside and outside gatherings, including church services, were forbidden, new and more flexible forms of the Eucharistic meal were developed in the Luther parish in Riga, the largest parish in the Latvian Evangelical Lutheran Church with 3,222 active parish members on December 31, 2020.

Until the pandemic, Holy Communion was part of the Sunday service; wine was distributed from a communal cup, and wafers were placed in the communicant's mouth by the person distributing the communion. In May 2020, the parish introduced an option for people to visit the church and organized a special individual way of receiving Holy Communion. Every Sunday from 12:00 noon until 2:00 pm, the church was open, musicians performed music, the pastor was standing at a table placed in front of the altar, and when people approached it, the pastor set out a single-use dish with bread and wine. The suggestion was that people should not stay in the church for more than 15 minutes. Every week, a worship service was videotaped so that the congregation could watch together on Sunday from 11:00 am to 12:00 noon on Zoom or at any time on YouTube. During the two hours' time-window on Sundays, there were about 50–70 people that came to receive communion, about 2–3 times less than the usual number of the communicants before the pandemic. These 1–3-minute long meditative moments of being together consisted of a brief greeting, a short exchange of a couple of words, a blessing, and a goodbye. This form of individual distribution gave a stronger sense of community and interpersonal resonance between the communicant and the pastor than before, but there were less opportunities for people to meet and communicate between themselves, though it did occasionally happen because there usually were no more than 10–15 people in the church. This form required great motivation, extra time, and energy. For many, it was a family event, possibly part of a Sunday road trip that was combined with a moment in the church building. Holy Communion became part of *something else*, not part of the usual in-person church service.

However, the real question is not so much about the distribution of Holy Communion that would suit the reality of the pandemic, but how much the Holy Communion format that had been used so far is still relevant, even for the existing parish members. During the pandemic, the interest in Holy Communion dropped significantly compared to the number of communicants before the pandemic. However, if before the pandemic video sermons were watched about 70–100 times, then during the pandemic that number grew to a constant 300–400 and more. Realizing that the digital means of communicating the gospel are here to stay and they have to be developed, the Luther parish is asking how to organize parish life so that digital access could be in balance with that which can be experienced only in person.

The task of practical theology is to model possible models of church work in the near future and to invite existing church activists to reflect on them and confront themselves with different and new ideas of how the church can express itself. One approach is to adapt the content and form of traditional face-to-face worship to the new human habits created by the COVID time, creating one common face-to-face and online format. But a more radical approach would be to evaluate the ability of the face-to-face format of worship to be the still dominant form of gospel communication and to transform it by creating entirely new digital models of the Holy Communion meal. These could serve each member of the digital community individually, while they are outside a particular space, in a remote communion of word and sacrament, both online but also outside a particular time – participating in a pre-recorded form of worship in which a communion of receiving, seeing, hearing the gospel and also the consecration of Holy Communion emerges. In this way, Holy Communion would no longer be tied to time and space, and a new, until now non-existent form of parish and church would emerge, more in tune with the habits, spiritual needs, self-understanding, and sense of reality of contemporary people. Today's challenges for the church and the church can be compared to the situation at the end of the Soviet era, when the church in Latvia was no longer able to fulfill its tasks and was in an existential crisis, facing new, as yet unknown tasks that would be important not only for the small and dwindling number of loyal members, but for the whole society, characterized by an enormous spiritual thirst and longing. It challenged us to think differently about the church and the congregation to develop new models and perspectives that are equally relevant to the transformation processes in the church today – processes that the post-doctoral project ""Succeeding in the sustainable and integrated development of society in the context of the 'Rebirth and Renewal' movement."[16] is exploring.

10 In-Depth Analysis Example No. 2: Riga Evangelical Parish (LELCW)

Parishes belonging to the Latvian LELCW are found in almost all the continents; they have followed a variety of practices regarding Holy Communion. Here, we will examine one of the LELCW parishes in Latvia to give an example of how the Eucharist was celebrated in the Latvian Lutheran church during the time of remote services.

When the pandemic restrictions started in Latvia in March 2020, the parish moved its services completely online. They took place on Zoom; parishioners and pastors joined from their homes; the church building was not used at this time. The order of the service changed as well; it was simplified and less responsive, many liturgical elements were abandoned, the communal singing was not practically feasible either. This small parish (about 80 people) had about 20–25 parishioners and guests in attendance. The parishioners testified that getting together on screen gave them a feeling of intimacy and even more direct contact among themselves. A new tradition was developed: to have a chat and share personal news before and after the service.

In the remote format of the service, Holy Communion was at first not celebrated. The parishioners did not ask to organize a Eucharistic service. However, following a suggestion by the pastor, the parish council agreed to celebrate a remote Holy Communion. On the first occasion at Easter 2021, this common meal was cautiously called Agape in case somebody could not accept this sort of remote communion. Encouraged by the widely used practice elsewhere in LELCW, the Riga Evangelical Lutheran parish later decided to celebrate communion online when everybody prepared his or her own bread and wine that would be consumed during the service.[17] The feedback of the parish in Riga was positive; one parishioner commented afterwards: "If God is everywhere, God is with me online as well." Until then, the words of consecration are said only by the pastor, but thinking about the development of hybrid services, the parishioners will also be invited to join in saying these words. That would be the way to develop the horizontal relationships in the Holy Communion liturgy where there is more than one person responsible for elements of the Eucharist. In its own way, it is also a reminder about the priesthood of all believers for the parishioners. Hybrid services leave their mark on the liturgy, which is simplified during the service the pastor always faces the parish, namely the camera, during the consecration of the Eucharist.

It is clear that in the future, the parish will be developing and improving the form of hybrid services, allowing people to gather both in person and remotely, celebrating the Eucharist in church and at their screens. That will provide the community of the parishes with new challenges to unite both the "visible" and the "invisible" parish.

11 Conclusion

The results of the survey and the analysis of the experiences in two different Lutheran parishes in Riga show that the COVID-19 pandemic has affected Holy Communion and the liturgy of church services on temporary and also more permanent levels. In this section, we will summarize our observations on the practice of Holy Communion, focusing our attention to its accessibility, location, time, and type.

First, with regard to its *accessibility* and *location*, we conclude that COVID-19 restrictions on social gatherings definitely affected the celebration of Holy Communion. There was considerable flexibility in the practice by different parishes and all surveyed parishes adjusted to the regulations. There was no particular resistance to the new rules; at least during the interviews, these objections were not raised. We can also see that not all parishes found new solutions and some of them ceased to celebrate Holy Communion. Smaller parishes were mostly affected negatively, they were already struggling before the COVID-19 crisis.

Other parishes were affected as far as the accessibility was concerned, depending on the restrictions on gathering. It could be observed that pastors and parish members made an extra effort to ensure that Holy Communion was accessible to those who could visit the parish. In the ELCL, there was no serious discussion about celebrating the Eucharist remotely, likely not because of organizational difficulties but rather because of theological decisions. The discussions on the questions about the Eucharist within the ELCL reviewed in this article show that there was an important emphasis on the way the sacrament was administered. It remained an exclusive prerogative of pastors, displaying deep reverence toward the elements. This has led to the lack of discussion about making Holy Communion accessible remotely. Such theology was not as prevalent in the LELCW, which is why remote celebration of the Eucharist was possible within its context. The abovementioned example from the online celebration of the Eucharist in the Riga Evangelical parish shows a new type of accessibility. People could participate in worship services and the Eucharist without going to church. However, a difference was also manifest between those churches with people who have digital skills and resources and those who do not, mostly depending on people's age. With regard to the location, the main place for celebrating Holy Communion in Latvia was still the church building. Consecration outside of it was practiced only in exceptional cases.

With regard to the *time* and *type* of Holy Communion, we have to conclude that it happened during a regular service or the time of its distribution was connected with the service, for example, on Sundays after the service where it was consecrated. The official directive to offer communion with intinction was not followed in every parish. It is interesting to see that, in the parishes where it was offered, communicants preferred the individual Eucharist to that of intinction. In light of that, one could say that they preferred the tradition of two elements to the communal aspect of a gathering at the altar. We think it is connected to the emphasis on the vertical communion during Holy Communion, which has dominated the ELCL parishes before, while the celebration of gathering of the people or the horizontal dimension is secondary. Also, celebrating Holy Communion with two elements is an essential part of the Lutheran identity for many parishioners.

In general, it can be said that Holy Communion was one of the most physical activities during this time. One can see that both pastors and parishioners made considerable efforts for the Eucharist to happen. It gained a new meaning as a physical activity because, for example, in the parishes that practiced remote services, many people drove to the church only to receive the communion. This physical dimension still played an important role.

Notes

1 Brodd,Theologien im Luthertum, 253.
2 Ibid., 249.
3 Erno, Luterāņu teoloģija Latvijā, 2.
4 Sildegs, Theology in the Ghetto, 126–128.
5 Talonen, *Baznīca Staļinisma žņaugos*, 23.
6 Vanags, Atjaunosim, 221.
7 Conference materials "Practice of the Lord's Supper in the ELCL", December 18, 1996.
8 Ibid.
9 Apparently, it refers to the theology of Thomas Aquinas who saw a symbolic meaning of Christ's suffering in the separation of blood from the body. STh III, q.

78, a.3, ad 7. Conference materials "Practice of the Lord's Supper in the ELCL, December 18, 1996.
10 Conference materials "Practice of the Lord's Supper in the ELCL", December 18, 1996.
11 Parish, The Absence of Presence.
12 Source: Privately conducted interview.
13 In many Latvian parishes there is a practice of the absolution being proclaimed by laying-on of hands either at the beginning of the service after the confession or before the distribution of the communion during the Eucharistic liturgy.
14 Aivars Gusevs, *LELB baznīcas gadagrāmata 2021* (Rīga: IHTIS, 2021), 220.
15 This practice was in Umurga, Sāti, Užava, Tukums, Vecsaule, Mērsrags, Vecsaule and Bauska.
16 "Panākumspēja sabiedrības ilgtspējīgai un integrālai attīstībai kustības "Atdzimšana un atjaunošanās" gadījuma kontekstā" (Nr.1.1.1.2/VIAA/3/19/498), a research project within the University of Latvia and Postdoc Latvia event "Pēcdoktorantūras pētniecības atbalsts."
17 There was an organized discussion for the LELCW pastors on May 4, 2021 where the majority of the attendants supported this sort of practice for a remote Holy Communion. The remote Eucharist was compared to the healing of the women with hemorrhages in Mark 5:25–34 where she touched Jesus' clothes, a "remote" touching of Jesus.

Works Cited

Brodd, Sven-Erik. "Eucharistische Theologien im Luthertum: ekklesiologische und sakramententheologische Perspektiven," *IKZ* 93 (2003): 249–265.

Erno, Jānis. *Luterāņu teoloģija Latvijā pasaules teoloģijas domas kontekstā (1983–1991)*. Bachelor thesis, Faculty of Theology, University of Latvia, 2009.

Gusevs, Aivars. "LELB draudžu statistika 2019.gads," *LELB baznīcas gadagrāmata* 2021. Rīga: Ihtis, 2021, 241–243.

Conference materials "Practice of the Lord's Supper in the ELCL" ("Svētā Vakarēdiena prakse LELB"), December 18, 1996, file "*Baznīcas Virsvalde 1996*", ELCL archive.

Parish, Helena. "The Absence of Presence and the Presence of Absence: Social Distancing, Sacraments, and the Virtual Religious Community during The Covid-19 Pandemic," *Religions 2020*, June 3, 2020, https://doi.org/10.3390/rel11060276 (accessed March 16, 2021).

Sildegs, Uģis. *Theology in the Ghetto: The Life, Work, and Theology of Nikolajs Plāte (1915–1983), Pastor and Theologian of the Evangelical Lutheran Church of the Latvian SSR*. University of Helsinki. Faculty of Theology. Helsinki: Unigrafia, 2017.

Talonen, Jouko. *Baznīca Staļinisma žņaugos: Latvijas Evaņģēliski luteriskā baznīca padomju okupācijas laikā no 1944. līdz 1950. gadam*. Rīga: Luterisma mantojuma fonds, 2009.

The Summa theologica of Saint Thomas Aquinas. Translated by Fathers of the English Dominican Province; revised by Daniel J. Sullivan, Chicago: Encyclopaedia Britannica, 1952.

Vanags, Jānis. "Atjaunosim savu draudžu dievgalda piederumus un tradīcijas!," *Baznīcas gadagrāmata 1999*. Rīga: Ihtis, 1999.

7 Ritual Reinvention and the Celebration of the Eucharist in Times of Crises

Biblical and Contemporary Perspectives

Korinna Zamfir

1 Introduction

This contribution started as a response to the crisis triggered by the SARS-CoV-2 pandemic, which has caused significant suffering due to the disease itself and the loss of loved ones, as well as frustration among practicing believers because of the restrictions implemented to prevent the spread of the infection. The interplay of these factors limited conventional worship in all Christian denominations, affecting the celebration of the Eucharist/the Lord's Supper. During the lockdown, in-person celebrations in churches became impossible. Later, constraints on gatherings remained in place, and social/physical distancing was required. Others experienced infection-related anxiety. Consequently, for about two years, the sacred space was (almost) out of reach. Reactions varied from fear to frustration and anger, to resignation and fatigue, to spiritual hunger and longing for alternatives. In several communities, the crisis was perceived as a challenge to overcome difficulties and create new ways of spiritual sharing and even experimenting with new forms of Eucharistic celebration where physical distance was overcome by online communication.

Meanwhile the fifth wave of the pandemic receded (before a new surge), but a new and even more terrible crisis emerged with the war against Ukraine. This challenged once again customary ways of worshipping and celebrating the Eucharist. Under the constant shelling of cities, due to curfews but also destruction, churches became again inaccessible. Believers of different denominations moved to underground shelters, from basements to metro stations, to hold liturgies and prayers.[1] On Easter 2022, online broadcasts of the liturgy were organized. Some churches continued to regularly broadcast Sunday services online.

Thus, while the challenges of the pandemic seemed to belong to the past, the new crisis in the shape of the war proved that religious communities and scholars of religion have to be ready to find responses, to adapt celebrations, in order to protect human life, to think of alternative rites carrying the same significance and provide spiritual comfort, so precious in any crisis.

The responses of theologians and church leaders to questions regarding the meaningfulness, validity, and efficacy of broadcasted or narrowcast

DOI: 10.4324/b22930-9

worship during the pandemic largely varied.[2] Opinions commonly focused on the shortcomings of such celebrations. I will argue instead that times of crises require creative solutions that take into account the reality and adapt the celebration of the Eucharist to the changed circumstances, using available means of communication to establish communion. Rites in which participants communicate through narrowcasting can become effective alternatives that allow genuine celebration in times of crises when physical participation is impossible.

This may require rethinking the concept of sacred space and developing a theological notion of sacred virtuality. To this end, I briefly explore two historical examples of the process of ritual transference of meaning: the crystallization of the *Seder* and the invention of the Eucharistic meal. In both cases, rites were adapted to the changed circumstances, and a theological concept (remembrance) was applied to transcend temporal and spatial distance from the foundational events. Subsequently, I turn to the notion of virtuality and argue that virtual celebrations should be seen as a new liturgical opportunity and theological challenge. Virtual participation refers here to situations when members of the community are not physically present in the church but share in worship and in the eucharistic celebration via narrowcasting platforms, which allow real time interaction, engaging in readings, prayers and chant, and even individual communion through gifts consecrated online. (I have in mind here the Catholic and Anglo-Catholic Eucharistic celebration.) This possibility involves, not unlike the invention of the *Seder* and that of the early Eucharistic meal, a reinvention of the rites and a new understanding of sacred space, based on a new, positive concept of virtuality. Sacred virtuality expresses the conviction that divine power (*virtus*) overcomes physical distance, being effective even in digital environments.

2 Reinventing the Rites

Rites celebrate and actualize the foundational events of religious communities and allow members to define and preserve their (collective) identity. In times of crises, however, certain essential rites may no longer be performed in long-established ways or cannot be performed at all. Under such circumstances, a reinvention of the rites enables the religious community to survive the crisis, generates hope, and opens new paths towards the future.

One such example was the Passover celebration in the aftermath of the first Jewish War. The war culminated in the destruction of the Temple in 70 CE, depriving the Jewish community of core elements of the cult, the sacrificial rites. The challenges of the war cannot be overestimated. As New Testament scholars, we often write and teach about the Jewish wars in a detached manner, perhaps even validate the rule of Rome in Judaea, Roman imperial concerns and military campaigns. But the tragic experience of the war waging once again in Europe, leading to the devastation of entire cities, to the destruction of churches and to scores of refugees forced to leave behind their entire life reminds us how disheartening a war can be. It also leads to a deeper understanding of the crisis ensuing from the loss of the Second Temple. From a religious perspective, these events led, among others, to a radical reconsideration of the celebration of the *Pesach*, the magnitude of which can hardly be overemphasized. While before the war the celebration was bound to the temple and involved sacrificial rites, the *Passover Seder* replaced these rites with a ritual meal celebrated in the family. Changes were thus twofold. The sacred space par excellence was replaced with the private space of the household, and dramatic rites were slimmed down to a cultic meal. However, due to the symbolic meaning assigned to specific foods and gestures, this ritual meal eventually became a core element of Jewish identity, expressing the same theological message of divine salvation. Soon, it became equivalent in importance to the sacrifices that could no longer be performed.

Sources from the Second Temple period do not mention the *Seder*. Aside the foundational biblical passages (Exod 12–13; Deut 16), which refer to the meal, Second Temple texts evoke the Passover/the Feast of the Unleavened, usually emphasizing sacrifices, without a detailed description of the rites celebrated at table. In the theological interpretation of the Passover, memory plays an important role.

Jubilees 49 (2nd cent. BCE) refers to sacrificing and eating the Passover lamb, drinking wine (49:1, 6, 9), and eating the unleavened bread (49:22). The text also connects the *Pesach* to the temple (49:16–17, 21).[3] The prohibition to eat outside the sanctuary indicates a shift from an earlier domestic celebration (probably following the Josianic Reform), a habit that most likely continued to be observed.[4] Remembrance is emphatic (49:1–2, 6).

A certain adaptation to specific circumstances (in the diaspora) surfaces already in Philo. Theologically, the Passover meal, as recollection and thanksgiving for the deliverance from Egypt,[5] has a marked spiritual dimension. Allegorically, the festival and its rites signify spiritual purification and a passage transcending bodily desires. As opposed to symposiasts, those who partake in the meal (συσσίτια) do not come together to gratify their appetites by indulging in meat and wine but to celebrate with prayers and hymns.[6] Philo does not connect the sacrifices to the temple and the priesthood. At this festival, Philo writes, all people offer sacrifices (θύουσι πανδημεί); during the time, every house receives the character and dignity of the temple (σχῆμα ἱεροῦ καὶ σεμνότητα).[7] Locating the rites in the domestic space is remarkable because, in Philo's time, the temple was still standing and sacrifices were performed in its precincts. But since not all diaspora Jews could observe an annual pilgrimage to Jerusalem, they expectedly did celebrate the Passover with a ritual meal in a household setting, possibly following domestic sacrifices.[8] (Philo never mentions the temple in Leontopolis. This suggests that for the Alexandrian diaspora, it was not seen as a significant alternative to the temple in Jerusalem.)[9]

Interestingly, although writing in the aftermath of the Jewish War, Josephus does not shed light on the attempts to make sense of the Passover when the temple no longer exists.[10] In two passages of the *Antiquities*, he emphasizes the renewal of the celebration in the temple during Hezekiah and Josiah and focuses on the sacrifices,[11] but it does not allude to the challenges of his time.

It will be rabbinic Judaism to reinvent the Passover meal and develop the *Seder* in response to the crisis following the destruction of the temple.[12] *Pesachim* 10 is the earliest witness.[13] This reinvention construed an accessible and full-fledged celebration of the Pesach even in the absence of sacrificial rites.[14] In the process, the unleavened bread and the ritual consumption of other foods (e.g., the *charoset*, the bitter herbs, or cooked food), and the accompanying gestures and words (lifting and naming the foods), became equivalent to the sacrifices and to eating the lamb.[15] Baruch Bokser has described this development as 'transference': during religious crises, the significance of lost sacred institutions or rites is transferred to other rituals. When the objects of the transfer of meaning – the temple and the associated rituals (the sacrifices) – become inaccessible or no longer exist, the community ascribes a similar meaning to alternative rites; the lost rite is substituted by another.[16]

Remembrance has a crucial role in this process: God's liberating intervention is brought into the present; it becomes a personal experience in every generation (Exod 13:8). Thus, temporal and physical distance from the foundational events is transcended, and the memory of the divine intervention grounds believers' future hope in times of crises (including oppression and war).[17]

The invention of the Eucharistic celebration also emerged (at least in part) in response to religious challenges through a process of ritual transference. The earliest communities of Jewish Christ-believers were compelled to (re-) define their identity and their rites in response to growing alienation from the group to which they had belonged, doubled by the same tragic experience of the war and the loss of the temple. The spread of the Christ-cult outside the community of Israel also contributed to the need to rethink older rites and create new ones. In the process, the remembrance of Jesus' Last Supper and death in the Eucharistic meal became a foundational rite, both in continuity and in discontinuity with the Passover meal. The idea that rites were bound to the Temple in Jerusalem also had to be reconsidered.

The earliest witness (1 Cor 11:23–26) does not address the nature of Jesus' Last Supper but links it to his passion and death. Yet earlier in the epistle (5:7–8), Paul associates Jesus' death with the sacrifice of the paschal lamb (τὸ πάσχα ἡμῶν ἐτύθη Χριστός) and invites believers to celebrate with unleavened bread (ἐν ἀζύμοις).[18] The celebration and the unleavened bread acquire a metaphorical-ethical sense. At the same time, at least typologically, Paul associates Jesus' death with the Pesach and the Feast of the Unleavened.[19] The sacrificial death of Christ becomes the new Passover of his followers, remembered during a ritual meal. This connection becomes explicit in the Synoptic Gospels. The Last Supper is Jesus' Passover meal,[20] which prefigures his passage through death to life. Thus, Jesus' last meal, the origin of the Eucharistic celebration, is construed both in continuity with the Pesach, in relation with the exodus and the covenant, [21] and as its reinterpretation. (This assessment stands regardless of the question whether the Last Supper was indeed a Passover meal.) The narratives create a cultic etiology with theologically and ritually significant gestures and words.[22] These ground the shared identity of Christ-believers by adopting and reimagining the categories of table fellowship, remembrance, and thanksgiving. In the process, remembrance, understood as an actualizing evocation (*anamnesis*) of the foundational events of Jesus' life, death, and resurrection, plays a major role.

3 Reinventing Sacred Space

The reinvention of the rites went together with the reinvention of sacred space. In the Hebrew Bible, sacred space may be the intangible setting of theophanies (Exod 3:1–5; 19:11–13), or more frequently, a sacred precinct properly speaking, the exclusive abode of JHVH, the temple, or the strictly secluded Holy of Holies, separated from the profane and inaccessible for common humans (Exod 26:31–34; Lev 16:2; cf. Heb 9:3, 7).[23] The importance of the temple increased with the Josianic Reform. However, following its destruction in 586 BCE and once more in 70 CE, Judaism was compelled to reconsider the question of sacred space.

The Babylonian period led to a broader, universal understanding of the presence of JHVH, no longer bound to Jerusalem and the temple.[24] Surely, after its reconstruction during the Persian period, the temple in Jerusalem retained its major significance. The impact of the two temples in the Egyptian diaspora, that of Elephantine under the Persian rule and of Leontopolis in the Ptolemaic and early Roman period, was rather limited both geographically and symbolically, and they never attained the significance of the temple in Jerusalem in the collective imaginary.[25]

As seen earlier, Philo accommodated the notion of sacred space by including the private home as venue of the Passover celebration. Through a transferal of meaning, he assigned the ritual significance of the temple to the domestic space.[26]

A more radical reconsideration of the sacred space occurred after 70 CE.[27] The survival of Judaism following the loss of the temple indicates a remarkable ability to adapt to new circumstances.[28] Nonetheless, the numerous references to the temple in the Mishna are puzzling, as they preserved its memory in its absence. This remembrance, just as the study of the sacrificial laws, probably worked as a replacement ritual, amounting perhaps to a virtual performance of the sacrifices.[29] To be sure, while the memory of the temple survived over the following centuries in texts and images, after 70 CE no other sacred space was established to replace it.[30]

Early Christ-believers were also challenged by the loss of the temple. The tearing of the temple curtain (Mark 15:38 par., cf. Heb 10:20) was probably a hint to a shift in the understanding of the sacred space following its devastation in 70 CE. For Jewish Christ-believers, this crisis required both a practical accommodation to the new situation and a theoretical reflection on what the loss of the temple meant. The temple imagery persists in the New Testament, but except for Acts, where the temple has a major role, and in John, the metaphor refers to the community (1 Cor 3:16–17; 6:16; Eph 2:21), the body of believers inhabited by the Spirit (1 Cor 6:19), the person of Jesus (John 2:19, 21) or the heavenly sanctuary (Heb, Rev). In fact, earliest communities of Christ-followers were lacking distinct sacred spaces for about two centuries.[31] The developing rites were hosted in private spaces or other, quite often prophane locations.[32] Thus, at its inception, the religious practice of the Christ-cult was not connected to a sacred space. It was only later that Christian churches carried further the distinction between the foremost sacred space, the sanctuary, and the nave, the place of common believers. Physical barriers – the iconostasis in the East, rails in the West – then reinforced this demarcation of sacred space.

Far from claiming the irrelevance of sacred space, these considerations instead posit the need to reconsider its importance and expand its definition. In various crises, when rites cannot be performed in such spaces, religious communities adapt and find ways to celebrate major rites pertaining to their identity elsewhere. This is the lesson taught by Jewish and early Christian communities. I will return to the topic on the margin of the notion of sacred virtual space.

4 Sacred Virtuality and Virtual Sacred Space

With the restrictions imposed during the pandemic, requiring social (or rather physical) distancing, several solutions were experimented as alternatives to face-to-face worship: from recorded or live-streamed services on television or social media to narrowcast Eucharistic celebrations on platforms like Zoom or Microsoft Teams.[33] While the former option meant watching the celebrant perform the rites alone or with a few people attending but without the possibility to interact,[34] the latter had the advantage of a real-time interactive experience. Besides listening to readings and the sermon, this could include a form of virtually shared Eucharistic table fellowship where the celebrant pronounced the words of consecration/institution over both the gifts placed before him (or her) and the bread and wine prepared by each participant in his/her own domestic space.[35]

Such practices, welcomed by many, have raised theological-philosophical debates regarding the validity of a Eucharistic celebration in the virtual space, more broadly about the value of virtual reality. The question is whether virtual reality, specifically communication and interaction in the virtual space through the mediation of narrowcasting platforms, can acquire the genuine personal character needed for participating effectively in the liturgy. Implicitly, this involves the question of whether the virtual space or environment can become a different kind of sacred space. Ultimately, can rites performed by a celebrant in one location, in which participants communicate through simultaneous narrowcasting, become effective alternative rites that allow genuine celebration in times of crises when physical participation is impossible?

Virtual reality is a much-debated concept, both on account of its meaning and its philosophical implications. It involves a physical (sensory) and mental immersion in a virtual world, in a computer-simulated medium, in a world that is either not directly present or imagined, by means of a computer-generated interface.[36] Physical/sensory and mental immersion convey the perception of being present and engaged in this environment. While physical reality is perceived first-hand, in experiencing virtual reality, direct sensory stimuli coming from physical objects are replaced or augmented through computer-based sensory stimulation. Immersion also involves the ability to interact with(in) the virtual environment. Virtual reality creates thus a collaborative digital space where several users can interact with each other, [37] "an immersive, interactive, computer-generated space."[38] Furthermore, virtual reality overcomes physical distance and produces significant effects – an important aspect for our topic.

Virtual reality has found numerous applications in science and education, in fields as diverse as medicine, manufacturing industries, urban planning, aeronautics, communication, psychology, as well as entertainment, and many other domains. To highlight only one, telesurgery is among the most notable achievements, attesting the capacity of virtual reality to overcome distance: the surgeon performs remote interventions on patients located elsewhere.[39] Thus, through a virtual medium, remarkable tangible effects occur, conceivable previously only through physical involvement.

Outside professional circles, the concept of virtual reality is usually met with suspicion, notably from a philosophical perspective. It is understood as the opposite of the real, of sense-perceptible reality, or at least of significantly lesser value. Furthermore, virtual reality is disparaged as artificial as opposed to the natural. Communication and interaction in the virtual environment are mediated and do not allow for immediate (apparently solely genuine) personal encounters that would require physical presence and contact.

Against the view that it would be fake or illusional, David Chalmers argues that virtual reality or "digital reality" is genuine reality, and the objects within it (virtual objects) are real, as they are made of digital processes, just as physical objects are made up of atoms and subatomic particles (ultimately quarks).[40] Moreover, Chalmers argues, virtual reality is Reality+: as an augmented reality, it is in some cases even better than ordinary reality.[41] (Chalmers defines his view as virtual realism.)[42]

Addressing the issue of worship in the virtual space, C. Andrew Doyle agrees with Chalmers that objects and persons in virtual reality are real, not illusory, as they are rooted in physical matter and physical processes. Yet, unlike Chalmers, he argues that they are substantially different from physical objects or persons, being merely digital representations of the former.[43] Through virtual media, we "perceive a very real moment from a very real representation communicated through very real physical matter," but not the totality of the event.[44] Virtual reality is a mediated reality. Therefore, Doyle allows that virtual worship may be significant and has some efficacy from a missiological perspective. However, broadcasting distorts the information.[45] Ultimately, the limitations of virtual worship are not compatible with a full Eucharistic celebration. Responding to Chalmers' view that virtual reality is genuine because participants are consciously present, make conscious choices, and act, Doyle accuses Chalmers of alleged brain theory reductionism, incompatible with Christian thinking because it reduces human consciousness to a network of neural transmissions in the brain.[46] He further claims that replicating and simulating the world through digital media would degrade inherent symbolic meanings as a sort of second-degree symbol void of significance. A virtual celebration would be a digitized simulation of the Eucharist, itself signifying the presence of Christ.[47]

Doyle's argument is strained and does not do justice to online celebrations. On the one hand, while admitting a certain reality to virtual objects, he does not underscore sufficiently the difference between a computer-generated virtual reality and the broadcasting or narrowcasting of events.[48] Broadcasting and, even more so, narrowcasting does not create a different reality, a computer-generated virtual world. Although physical proximity is not achievable, real-time participation in a narrowcast, interactive liturgical service truly transcends distance. This involves a real, albeit mediated, presence and engagement, not a digitized simulation. Furthermore, the most essential senses – sight and hearing, i.e., elements of our physical dimension – participate. This leads to a genuine sensory and mental immersion in the liturgical celebration, where real communication and communion occur.

Doyle's argument that virtual reality is mediated, thus not genuine, also obscures the fact that all forms of perception and interaction are mediated, even when a person or object is physically present. Perception is mediated through complex processes in the central nervous system. Sense-perception is a neural, electric and chemical simulation of the physical objects. There is no such thing as immediate, unmediated, and thus allegedly undistorted perception. Additionally, connections between primary sensitive-sensorial and associative cortical areas evoke memories of formerly acquired knowledge. Remembrance has thus the power to bring past, long-elapsed events and experiences into the present, despite their physical distance. A strict distinction between in-person, apparently non-mediated, and online, mediated participation is therefore overstated.

Doyle challenges Chalmers' anthropology as reductionist (humans are allegedly reduced to mere consciousness) against a holistic, incarnational Christian anthropology, which values bodily existence.[49] It is beyond the purpose of this paper to examine Chalmers' anthropological views. However, the sensory immersion in virtual reality endows in fact participation with a physical, not purely mental, dimension. Leaving aside the fact that Christian anthropology has hardly been consistently holistic, it cannot be argued that the bodily dimension is eliminated in a synchronous virtual (online) participation in liturgy.

In addition, even at in-person celebrations, physical participation, as important as it may be, it is in fact subordinated to spiritual participation. In the latter, remembrance plays a significant role. Memory evokes and rites actualize the events of salvation history, which become accessible to participants not as physical perceptions but as spiritual experiences.

More importantly, however, while physical presence is obviously important, the genuineness and effectiveness of the liturgical celebration depend foremost on theological, not anthropological, aspects. As important as anthropological considerations are, ultimately it is divine agency that transcends temporal and spatial distance from past foundational events – the Lord's Supper, Christ's redeeming death on the cross, and the resurrection that overcomes death.

A particular question has emerged regarding the range within which divine action retains its effectiveness, more specifically the range of consecration, on which the validity and the efficacy of online Eucharists depends.[50] In response to such doubts, Richard Burridge rightly rejects "a mechanistic or quasi-magical interpretations" of the words of institution and emphasizes instead two significant theological factors: the intention of the celebrant and the epicletic dimension of consecration.[51] If intention embraces the elements (bread and wine) that the participants in a narrowcast liturgy have placed before them, visible to the celebrant on the screen, then physical distance cannot be an obstacle. More importantly, in Eucharistic celebration, the celebrant usually invokes the Holy Spirit upon the bread and wine so that they may become the body and blood of Christ.

Divine agency can in no way depend on the distance between the celebrant and those who participate through the interface of the screen. It would be extremely odd to claim that divine agency has spatial limits, considering the tangible effectiveness of human agency in telesurgery performed through virtual mediation.

We may therefore envisage a new, theological understanding of virtuality, relying on the notion of *virtus Dei*, the boundless, effective power of God, of the Holy Spirit, which transcends physical and temporal distance.[52] In this understanding, even in a digitally mediated environment, God works through the preaching of Scriptures, but also in the Eucharistic celebration proper. "Virtual" participation is not the opposite of "real" participation, but a particular manner of experiencing the power, the *virtus* of God.

This also involves the notion of a virtual sacred space, reflecting the conviction that not only the physical realm, but the digital world too belongs to the creation of God and is capable of becoming the place of divine presence and manifestation.[53]

This leads to a new experience of communion. Critics argue that online worship deprives believers of the sense of communion resulting from interactions with other participants.[54] In fact, narrowcast Eucharistic celebrations, if appropriately prepared, may allow a very similar experience of communion, and through the interactive character may even lead to a deeper personal involvement.[55]

5 Conclusions

Any religious community stands, on the one hand, in continuity with the faith and practice of earlier generations, with the foundational events of its past. On the other hand, crises and turning points in history raise challenges that demand creative responses. These may involve the reinvention of the rites and sacred spaces.

Reinvention presupposes a transference of meaning from rites and spaces no longer accessible to new rites and spaces. This was the case with Judaism after the destruction of the Second Temple. The meaning of sacrifices was transferred to symbolic gestures and words accompanying the *Seder*, a ritual meal celebrated in the domestic space.

The early followers of Jesus needed to respond to the death of their founding figure, the loss of the temple, and the gradual separation from Judaism. The memory of Jesus' Last Supper, interpreted as his Passover, sacrifice, and covenant, actualized in the Eucharistic meal, became a central rite that could be performed in the domestic space or even in profane venues.

Remembrance (*anamnesis*) played a crucial role in both cases, as it brought the foundational events into the present, overcoming temporal and spatial distance and creating a virtual, spiritual communion. These developments hold important lessons for contemporary crises (pandemics or wars) that may impact the performance of rites and prevent access to sacred space.

Digital technologies have provided previously unthinkable ways of interaction and have been used creatively during recent crises. Despite their limitations, broadcasted liturgies have provided comfort to many believers in difficult circumstances. More importantly, narrowcast, interactive liturgies have led to the emergence of novel ways of experiencing the limitless power (*virtus*) of God. A sort of ritual transference occurred. While physical sacred space was no longer available, a new, virtual sacred space emerged. Consecrating the elements and sharing in the Eucharistic meal through a digital medium expressed the conviction that the *virtus* of God cannot be limited by physical distance. The underlying assumption is not entirely different from that which grounded the concept of *anamnesis*: there is no distance, whether temporal or spatial, that God cannot transcend.

Critics may raise objections based on philosophical and anthropological arguments, some of which point indeed to the limits of celebrations in a virtual environment. But the ritual transference underlying the invention of the

Seder and the Eucharist demonstrates that openness to new ways of celebrating may be the only way to survive deep crises.

This is not to say that in-person celebration with a community assembled in sacred space is not preferable. But instead of complaining about limitations and restrictions and surrendering to frustration, communities of faith should discover and acknowledge new ways of celebrating and experiencing communion.

Notes

1 RISU: "*Priests Descend into Bomb Shelters*"; Bordoni, "*Ukrainian Priests*"; Church of England: "*Priest's Prayers for Peace*"; Lozano, "*Ukraine: Prayers*".
2 Broadcasting refers here to livestreaming religious services on television, radio or online, which can be followed but do not allow active engagement in the celebration. Narrowcasting involves platforms like Zoom or Microsoft Teams, through which believers are offered personal, real time, online interaction.
3 Vanderkam, *Jubilees*, 315–325.
4 Marcus, "Passover," 308–309.
5 The celebration is remembrance (ὑπόμνημα) and thanksgiving (χαριστήριον) for the deliverance from Egypt, an annual memorial of gratitude (εἰς εὐχαριστίας ὑπόμνησιν) for a singular event. Spec. leg. 2:145–148.
6 Spec. leg. 2:148. Actually, this polemical remark implicitly points to formal similarities with the Graeco-Roman symposium. Siegfried Stein had emphasized the influence of the symposium on the crystallization of the *Seder*: "Influence," 13–44. Baruch M. Bokser questions the impact of the symposium, beyond some formal similarities (*Origins*, 50–66). Philo contrasts Jewish festal commensality to heathen self-indulgence. Later, Tertullian will do the same with respect to the Eucharistic meal (*Apol.* 38–39).
7 Spec. leg. 2:145, 148.
8 Bokser thinks this was probably the case, but finds it difficult to prove (*Origins*, 54, 61). Jutta Leonhardt challenges the view that the ritual also involved sacrifices, because these had to be performed in the temple precincts. She argues, therefore, that Philo referred to the meal celebrated by pilgrims in Jerusalem (*Jewish Worship*, 32–33). Clemens Leonhard rejects the possibility in even stronger terms (*Jewish Pesach*, 33–35). However, in Philo there is no reference to Jerusalem. Jordan D. Rosenblum does not find it impossible that in exceptional cases sacrifices could be offered in the context of domestic celebration: "Home is Where the Hearth is?," 157–158. To be sure, this is how John M.G. Barclay (*Jews in the Mediterranean Diaspora*, 415), Federico M. Colautti (*Passover*, 232) and Marcus ("Passover", 309) interpret Philo.
9 Frey, "Temple," 187, 192, 194, 197.
10 This might be due to the apologetic character of his work. In the *Jewish War* he refers frequently to the Passover, but mostly in relation to events of the war (*Bell.* 2:10, 224, 280; 4:404; 5:99–100; 6:421–434). In the *Antiquities* he narrates historical events associated with the Passover (11:109–111; 17:213–215; 18:29–30, 90). He usually speaks of the Feast of the Unleavened, to which he connects the πάσκα secondarily, to refer to the feast or the sacrifices (*Ant.* 9:263–264; 11:109; 17:213: ἄζυμα [...] πάσκα δ᾽ ἡ ἑορτὴ καλεῖται ὑπόμνημα οὖσα τῆς ἐξ Αἰγύπτου ἀπάρσεως).
11 Aside the origins of the Passover (*Ant.* 2:312–313), he speaks of its restoration during Hezekiah (9:263–272) and its celebration under Josiah (10:70–73). See the

detailed discussion of Josephus by Colautti, *Passover in the Works of Josephus* (2002). He notes that Josephus is more permissive regarding the celebration of the Passover outside Jerusalem (ibid., 163, 232).

12 Bokser, *Origins*, 1–3, passim; Tabory, "History," 62–80; Yuval, "Easter and Passover," 98–124. Yuval argues that the *Seder* and the Passover Haggadah developed in response to the Christian reinterpretation of the *Pesach*, the narratives of the Last Supper, and the Eucharistic celebration. One cannot exclude reciprocal influences in the formative period of Christianity and Judaism, but Yuval's examples are not very convincing. David Golinkin rightly challenges Yuval's thesis ("Origins," 76–100).

13 For analyses, see Bokser, *Origins*, 14–28; Instone-Brewer, *Traditions*, 172–200 (distinguishing between pre- and post-70 traditions).

14 Bokser, *Origins*, 1–3, 28, 37–40, 49–50, 67, passim; Tabory, "History," 62–80; Yuval, "Easter and Passover," 99, 114.

15 See the detailed analysis of Bokser, *Origins*, 29–49, idem, "Ritualizing the Seder," 443–471.

16 *Origins*, 57–61 (following Neusner, *from Politics to Piety*).

17 Remembering the exodus kept hope alive during the Roman rule, salvation was appropriated by every generation, grounding the expectance of future redemption: Bokser, *Origins*, 25, 72–73, 75–80, 83–84; idem, "Ritualizing the Seder," 445.

18 Thiselton, *First Corinthians*, 405, 878–879; Marcus, "Passover," 371; Collins, *First Corinthians*, 214.

19 Jeremias, *Eucharistic Words*, 74; Conzelmann, *1 Korinther*, 126; Thiselton, *First Corinthians*, 873–874. Schrage prefers the Johannine chronology and interprets 1 Cor 5:7 typologically (*1 Kor 1,1–6,11*, 383, and *1 Kor 11,17–14,40*, 31, n. 466). The motif of the Passover lamb matches the metaphorical use of sacrificial terminology in Judaism and Christianity. Klawans, "Interpreting the Last Supper," 13–16.

20 For a discussion, see Jeremias, *Eucharistic Words*, 41–88; Gnilka, *Markus*, 243–248; Luz, *Matthäus*, 102 (not identical with the *Seder*); Donahue, Harrington, *Mark*, 398–399; Fiedler, *Matthäusevangelium*, 788; Marcus, "Passover," 303–324. Critical of the idea of a Passover meal: Alikin, *Earliest History*, 121–122; Weidemann, "Bundesblut," 56–98. Cautiously assessing the options: Kazen, "Sacrificial Interpretation," 477–502.

21 On the continuity with the Sinai-covenant: Fiedler, *Matthäusevangelium*, 390; pace Luz, *Matthäus*, 115. See also Klawans, "Interpreting the Last Supper," 15; Kazen, "Sacrificial Interpretation," 477–502.

22 Gnilka, *Markus*, 241; Luz, *Matthäus* 4, 95; Collins, *First Corinthians*, 428.

23 Obviously, the delineation of a distinct space – the temple or its inner chamber (the *naos* or *cella*), inhabited by the god(dess) – was common in Greek and Roman religion as well.

24 For the contribution of Ezekiel (without contesting the importance of the physical temple): Joyce, "On Earth as It Is in Heaven," 123–139. Chavel provides a different perspective: "Yahweh Become a Temple?," 103–122.

25 On the historical context and limited role of the temples of Elephantine and Leontopolis: Frey, "Temple," 171–203.

26 Bokser, *Origins*, 58.

27 Rendsburg, "Sacred Space", 15–49.

28 Rendsburg, "Sacred Space", 17.

29 Rendsburg, "Sacred Space", 21–22.

30 Rendsburg, "Sacred Space", 24–41.

31 This does not mean that early Christian conceptions of sacred space were topophobic (rightly, Hadley, "Early Christian Perceptions", 89–90).

32 Horrell, "Domestic Space," 349–369; Adams, *Earliest Christian Meeting Places*, 137–202; Kloppenborg, *Christ's Associations*, 104–105, 116–119.
33 Zipple, "Lessons".
34 Several other options, like the Eucharistic fast, the spiritual communion, the broadcasted solo celebration and communion, have been rightly criticized, because they excluded believers from communion. See Burridge, *Holy Communion*, 29–60.
35 Burridge, *Holy Communion*, 248–272.
36 I summarize here some of the features described by Sherman and Craig, *Understanding Virtual Reality*, 2002, and Chalmers, *Reality+*, 2022.
37 Sherman, Craig, *Understanding Virtual Reality*, 5–17.
38 Chalmers, *Reality+*, xix-xx, 12, 14.
39 The pioneering laparoscopic cholecystectomy performed by Marescaux and Gagner, both located in New York at Mount Sinai Medical Centre, on a patient hospitalized at the European Institute of Telesurgery in Strasbourg, in September 2001. Marescaux, Leroy, Gagner *et al.*, "Transatlantic Robot-Assisted Telesurgery", 379–380.
40 Chalmers, *Reality+*, 14, and further ch. 6 (What is Reality?).
41 Chalmers, *Reality+*, xviii, xxii, 108.
42 Chalmers, *Reality+*, 105–106.
43 Doyle, *Embodied Liturgy*, 8.
44 Doyle, *Embodied Liturgy*, 9.
45 Doyle, *Embodied Liturgy*, 9–10, 14.
46 Doyle, *Embodied Liturgy*, 11–12.
47 Doyle, *Embodied Liturgy*, 15–16. He applies Jean Baudrillard's notion of simulacra, of endless proliferations of images, of meaningless signs, media-created copies of reality, which obscure the truth, devoid the signs of their meaning, leading to the image taking precedence over reality. However, Baudrillard's nostalgia for an idealized (pre-)modern realm where the truth, the real was not (yet) obscured, his quasi-apocalyptic perspective is not really helpful for this discussion. For a critique of Baudrillard: Sokal and Bricmont, "Jean Baudrillard," 147–153; Norris, *Uncritical Theory*, 1992; Kellner, "Jean Baudrillard".
48 He speaks at a certain point of "an AI priest that makes Eucharist for avatar communicants" (*Embodied Liturgy*, 13). Furthermore, he focuses on "watching a prerecorded liturgy" that "diminishes the participatory character, the interactions with other participants" (ibid., 31).
49 Doyle, *Embodied Liturgy*, 10–15.
50 Burridge, *Holy Communion*, 258.
51 Burridge, *Holy Communion*, 258–259.
52 The Vulgate renders thus the power of God. Also *Deus virtutum*, God of Hosts, in Psalms; Wisdom, as "vapor ... virtutis Dei" and emanation of the glory of divine omnipotence (Wis 7:25). In the NT, it is manifest in the gospel message (Rom 1:16, 20), in the message of the cross (1 Cor 1:18); also the *virtus Altissimi* (Luke 1:35). *Virtus Dei* is a notion used in Western theology for the power of God since the second century: Tert., *Adv. Marc.* 4:26 (cf. Luke 11:20); Aug., *Trin.* 3:9:18; 3:7:12; Ambr. *In Luc.* 7:93 (the Holy Spirit), cf. Chrupcała, *Everyone*, 254–257.
53 Burridge, *Holy Communion*, 267; Salurante *et al.*, "A Virtual Sacred Space," 144–146.
54 Doyle, *Embodied Liturgy*, 31, of watching a prerecorded liturgy; online services would deprive believers of the communion "with the saints of old." Yet, even at in-person worship, experiencing togetherness with long-gone people occurs in faith and spiritual communion, i.e., in a different kind of virtuality.
55 Burridge, *Holy Communion*, 271 (gathering, attending, communing in prayer and in the sacrament, and dispersing to everyday life); Zipple, "Lessons".

Bibliography

Adams, Edward, *The Earliest Christian Meeting Places – Almost Exclusively Houses?* London: Bloomsbury, 2013, 137–202.

Alikin, Valeriy A., *The Earliest History of the Christian Gathering: Origin, Development and Content of the Christian Gathering in the First to Third Centuries*, Leiden: Brill, 2010.

Barclay, John M.G., *Jews in the Mediterranean Diaspora: From Alexander to Trajan (323 BCE 117 CE)*, Berkley: University of California Press, 1996.

Bokser, Baruch, "Ritualizing the Seder," *Journal of the American Academy of Religion* 56.3 (1988): 443–471.

Bokser, Baruch M., *The Origins of the Seder: The Passover Rite and Early Rabbinic Judaism*, Berkley; Los Angeles: University of California Press, 1986.

Bordoni, Linda, "Ukrainian Priests to Celebrate Mass in Kyiv Bomb Shelters," *Vatican News* (27 February 2022), https://www.vaticannews.va/en/church/news/2022-02/major-archbishop-shevchuk-video-message-ukraine.html.

Burridge, Richard, *Holy Communion in Contagious Times: Celebrating the Eucharist in the Everyday and Online Worlds*, Eugene, OR: Wipf and Stock, 2022.

Chalmers, David J., *Reality+: Virtual Worlds and the Problems of Philosophy*, New York: W.W. Norton, 2022.

Chavel, Simeon, "Yahweh Become a Temple? MT Ezekiel 11:16 מִקְדָּשׁ מְעַט Revisited", in *Contextualizing Jewish Temples* (The Brill Reference Library of Judaism, 64), edited by Tova Ganzel and Shalom E. Holtz, Leiden: Brill, 2020, 103–122.

Chrupcała, Lesław Daniel, *Everyone Will See the Salvation of God: Studies in Lukan Theology*, Milano: Terra Santa, 2015.

Colautti, Federico M., *Passover in the Works of Josephus*, Leiden: Brill, 2002.

Collins, Raymond F., *First Corinthians* (SP 7), Collegeville, MN: Liturgical Press, 1999.

Conzelmann, Hans, *Der erste Brief an die Korinther* (KEK), Göttingen: Vandenhoeck & Ruprecht, 1981 (12th ed.).

Donahue, John R. and Daniel J. Harrington, *The Gospel of Mark* (SP 2), Collegeville, MI: Liturgical Press, 2002.

Doyle, C. Andrew, *Embodied Liturgy: Virtual Reality and Liturgical Theology in Conversation*, New York: Church Publishing, 2021.

Fiedler, Peter, *Das Matthäusevangelium* (ThKNT), Stuttgart: Kohlhammer, 2006.

Frey, Jörg, "Temple and Rival Temple – The Cases of Elephantine, Mt. Gerizim, and Leontopolis," in *Gemeinde ohne Tempel / Community Without Temple*, edited by Beate Ego, Armin Lange and Peter Pilhofer with Kathrin Ehlers (WUNT 118), Tübingen: Mohr Siebeck, 1999, 171–203.

Gnilka, Joachim, *Das Evangelium nach Markus: Mk 8,27 – 16,20* (EKK II/2), Zürich: Patmos; Neukirchen-Vluyn: Neukirchener, 1979.

Golinkin, David, "The Origins of the Seder," *Insight Israel* 6.8 (2006): 76–100.

Hadley James T., "Early Christian Perceptions of Sacred Spaces," *Revue de la culture matérielle* 80–81 (2014–2015): 89–107.

Horrell, David G., "Domestic Space and Christian Meetings at Corinth: Imagining New Contexts and the Buildings East of the Theatre," *New Testament Studies* 50 (2004): 349–369.

Instone-Brewer, David, *Traditions of the Rabbis from the Era of the New Testament: 2A. Feasts and Sabbaths: Passover and Atonement*, Grand Rapids, MI: Eerdmans, 2011, 172–200.

Jeremias, Joachim, *The Eucharistic Words of Jesus*, London: SCM, 1987 (7th ed.).

Josephus, *Jewish Antiquities*, vol. I (LCL 242), translated by Henry St. J. Thackeray; vol. IV: (LCL 326), translated by Ralph Marcus; vol. VII, translated by Ralph Marcus, Allen Wikgren (LCL 410); vol. VIII, translated by Louis H. Feldman (LCL 433), Cambridge, MA: Harvard University Press, 1930, 1937, 1963, 1965.

Josephus, *The Jewish War*, vol. I (LCL 203), vol. II (LCL 487), vol. III (LCL 210), translated by Henry St. J. Thackeray, Cambridge, MA: Harvard University Press, 1927–1928.

Joyce, Paul M., "On Earth as It Is in Heaven: Heavenly and Earthly Temple in Ezekiel 40–48", in *Contextualizing Jewish Temples* (The Brill Reference Library of Judaism, 64), edited by Tova Ganzel and Shalom E. Holtz, Leiden: Brill, 2020, 123–139.

Kazen, Thomas, "Sacrificial Interpretation in the Narratives of Jesus' Last Meal," in *The Eucharist – Its Origins and Contexts: Sacred Meal, Communal Meal, Table Fellowship in Late Antiquity, Early Judaism, and Early Christianity* I (WUNT 376), edited by David Hellholm and Dieter Sänger, Tübingen: Mohr Siebeck, 2017, 477–502.

Kellner, Douglas, "Jean Baudrillard", in *The Stanford Encyclopedia of Philosophy*, edited by Edward N. Zalta, (2020), https://plato.stanford.edu/archives/win2020/entries/baudrillard/.

Klawans, Jonathan, "Interpreting the Last Supper: Sacrifice, Spiritualization, and Anti-Sacrifice," *NTS* 48 (2002): 1–17.

Kloppenborg, John, *Christ's Associations: Connecting and Belonging in the Ancient City*, New Haven: Yale University Press, 2019.

Leonhard, Clemens, *The Jewish Pesach and the Origins of the Christian Easter: Open Questions in Current Research*, Berlin: Walter de Gruyter, 2006.

Leonhardt, Jutta, *Jewish Worship in Philo of Alexandria* (TSAJ 84), Tübingen: Mohr Siebeck, 2001.

Lozano, Maria, "Ukraine: Prayers in the Air Raid Shelter, Aid to the Church in Need," *Church in Need*, (3 March 2022), https://www.churchinneed.org/ukraine-prayers-in-the-air-raid-shelter/.

Luz, Ulrich, *Das Evangelium nach Matthäus 4: Mt 26–28* (EKK 1/4), Düsseldorf; Zürich: Benziger; Neukirchen-Vluyn: Neukirchener Verlag, 2002.

Marcus, Joel, "Passover and Last Supper Revisited," *NTS* 59 (2013): 303–324.

Marescaux, Jacques, Joel Leroy, Michel Gagner *et al.*, "Transatlantic Robot-Assisted Telesurgery," *Nature* 413 (2001): 379–380, https://doi.org/10.1038/35096636.

Neusner, Jacob, *From Politics to Piety: The Emergence of Pharisaic Judaism*, New York: Ktav, 1979 (2nd ed.).

Norris, Christopher, *Uncritical Theory: Postmodernism, Intellectuals & the Gulf War*, Amherst, MA: University of Massachusetts Press, 1992.

Philo, vol. VIII: *On the Special Laws, On the Virtues. On Rewards and Punishments* (LCL 341), vol. IX: *Every Good Man Is Free; The Contemplative Life; The Eternity of the World; Against Flaccus; Apology for the Jews; On Providence* (LCL 363), translated by Francis H. Colson, Cambridge, MA: Harvard University Press, 1939; 1941.

"Priests Descend into Bomb Shelters: Divine Liturgy in the Kyiv Metro," *Religious Information Service of Ukraine* (25 March 2022), https://risu.ua/en/priests-descend-into-bomb-shelters-divine-liturgy-in-the-kyiv-metro_n127678.

"Priest's Prayers for Peace from Ukrainian Bomb Shelter to lead BBC Radio Service," *Church of England* (4 March 2022), https://www.churchofengland.org/media-and-news/press-releases/priests-prayers-peace-ukrainian-bomb-shelter-lead-bbc-radio-service.

Rendsburg, Gary A., "Sacred Space in Judaism after the Temple," in *Sacred Space, Sacred Thread: Perspectives across Time and Traditions*, edited by John W. Welch and Jacob Rennaker, Eugene, OR: Wipf and Stock, 2019, 15–49.

Rosenblum, Jordan D., "Home is Where the Hearth Is? A Consideration of Jewish Household Sacrifice in Antiquity", in *"The One Who Sows Bountifully": Essays in Honor of Stanley K. Stowers* (Brown Judaic Studies), edited by Caroline Johnson Hodge, Saul M. Olyan, Daniel Ullucci, and Emma Wasserman, Providence, RI: Brown University, 2013, 153–163.

Salurante, Tony, David Kristanto, Malik Malik, Lewi Nataniel Bora, and Nelly Nelly, "A Virtual Sacred Space. Some Theological Considerations", in Adriadi Novawan *et al.*, *Proceedings of the 2nd International Conference on Social Science, Humanity and Public Health* (ICOSHIP 2021), (Advances in Social Science, Education and Humanities Research, 645), Amsterdam: Atlantis Press (Springer Nature), 2022, 144–146.

Schrage, Wolfgang, *Der Erste Brief an die Korinther: 1 Kor 1,1–6,11* (EKK VII/1); *1 Kor 11,17–14,40* (EKK VII/3), Zürich: Benzinger; Neukirchen-Vluyn: Neukirchener, 1991, 1999.

Sherman, William R. and Alan Craig, *Understanding Virtual Reality: Interface, Application, and Design*, San Francisco: Morgan Kaufmann, 2002.

Sokal, Alan and Jean Bricmont, "Jean Baudrillard", in idem, *Fashionable Nonsense: Postmodern Intellectuals' Abuse of Science*, New York: Picador, 1998, 147–153.

Stein, Siegfried, "The Influence of Symposia Literature on the Literary Form of the Pesah Haggadah," Journal of Jewish Studies 8 (1957): 13–44.

Tabory, Joseph, "Towards a History of the Paschal Meal", in *Passover and Easter: Origin and History to Modern Times* (Two Liturgical Traditions 5.), edited by Paul Bradshaw and Lawrence A. Hoffman, Notre Dame, IN: University of Notre Dame Press, 1999, 62–80.

Thiselton, Anthony C., *The First Epistle to the Corinthians: A Commentary on the Greek Text* (NIGTC), Grand Rapids, MI: Eerdmans, 2000.

Vanderkam, James C., *The Book of Jubilees* (CSCO 511; Scriptores Aethiopici 88), Leuven: Peeters, 1989, 315–325.

Weidemann, Hans-Ulrich, "'Dies ist mein Bundesblut' (Mk 14,24): Die markinische Abendmahlserzählung als Beispiel für liturgisch beeinflusste Transformationsprozesse," in *Aneignung durch Transformation: Beiträge zur Analyse von Überlieferungsprozessen im frühen Christentum: Festschrift für Michael Theobald* (HBS 74), edited by Wilfried Eisele, Christoph Schäfer, and Hans-Ulrich Weidemann, Freiburg: Herder, 2013, 56–98.

Yuval, Israel Y., "Easter and Passover as Early Jewish-Christian Dialogue," in *Passover and Easter: Origin and History to Modern Times* (Two Liturgical Traditions 5.), edited by Paul Bradshaw and Lawrence A. Hoffman, Notre Dame, IN: University of Notre Dame Press, 1999, 98–124.

Zipple, Jeremy, "Lessons from a Year of Online Liturgy at a Jesuit Parish in Belize," *America Magazine* (9 March 2021), https://www.americamagazine.org/faith/2021/03/09/belize-coronavirus-mass-worship-online-liturgy-jesuit-240183.

8 Isolation, Community, and Religious Identification

The Ritual World of Early Christian Imprisonment Letters

Soham Al-Suadi

1 Introduction

Paul is known to many readers as an apostle who founded communities and searches for optimal conditions to make social life possible. In this essay, Paul is described as an author who writes not only about community, but also about isolation to his readers. He addresses both issues primarily in a ritual context. The letters from the apostle's imprisonment, the so-called captivity letters, depict prison as a place which inevitably made the imprisoned think and talk about God. Not only the Epistle to the Philippians and the Epistle to Philemon, but also the Epistle to the Ephesians and the Epistle to the Colossians describe imprisonment from metaphorical, historical, and theological perspectives. Isolation is described in the Epistle to the Colossians by a narrow circle of intimates (Col 4:10–5), by the metaphor of death (Col 4:2–3) as well as by soteriological hope (Col 1:24–25)[1] being the sole hope of the prisoner. Although the letter to the Ephesians addresses a group in the first chapter, it decidedly adds isolation and loneliness, speaking on the committee of the citizenship of Israel and calling the readers strangers with regard to the covenants of the promise. Having no hope and being without God in the world are real experiences (Eph 2:12). The Epistle to Philemon also speaks metaphorically of Paul the prisoner (Phlm 1), only to add separation between Onesimus and his master in Philemon 15. Here, Paul is looking for a reason why Onesimus has been separated from his master for a time, so that he can subsequently be accepted forever as a beloved brother. In Philippians, Paul speaks of his bonds in the very first verse (Phil 1:14), mirroring the image he uses to express his courage by proclaiming the Word of God (Phil 1:20).

This introductory outlook on the topics of isolation, community, and religious identification in the captivity letters already reveals a diversity that deserves to be put into adequate context. This paper contextualizes the experiences described regarding ritual. The basis for this is the assumption that imprisonment is a temporary, socially constructed life situation that necessitates ritual behaviors due to the deprivation of freedom and social isolation. Studying rituals in a captive situation also touches on the field of the form of communication. Written or oral communication is characterized by

DOI: 10.4324/b22930-10

limitations, not only due to spatiality but also due to the differential or unresolved use of power. In academic debate, this communication is described as the "hidden transcripts." They are an essential component in various communication situations, which are examined in the case of prayer language in the captivity letters.

In previous publications, I have drawn closely on the ritual studies of Ronald Grimes, who investigates ritual in everyday contexts, and I will continue relating to his work.[2] Whether we are involved in ritualization is not for us to decide. We can only choose whether we are attentive or repressive to actions that surround us and from which we cannot escape.[3] I am convinced that in Grimes' theoretical approach, no distinction is made between everyday rituals and particular rituals. This is peculiar in the context of deprivation of liberty because deprivation of liberty establishes a normality beyond everyday life of the broad public. This is as true for metaphorical descriptions as it is for socio-historical descriptions. For Grimes, this human capacity becomes evident in ritualization, which, in turn, is the result of a "genetic culture" and in this respect has involuntary, unavoidable features. Any community or group accommodated to certain rituals will find immediate comfort in interaction.[4]

In the following three sections, I will turn to the captivity letters with Grimes' theory. First, under the assumption that ritual is a cultural experience that provides an agreement for comfort in social conditions, I will show the ritual imagery of imprisonment in the letters. Second, I will describe the tension between isolation and community in Pauline discourse and show what isolation and social distance mean to Paul. Third, I will understand ritualization as an expression of personal and collective experiences of crisis and explore the thesis that ritual aspects do not only stabilize community but also its opposite, isolation, and exclusion.

2 Pauline Voices on Isolation and Community

2.1 Rituals as Cultural Experiences in the Imprisonment Letters

Matthew Skinner explains that

> in most cases, biblical references to imprisonment do not denote separate and dedicated structures with fortifications and individual cells. Although many larger cities in the Roman Empire of the first century had discrete prison buildings used primarily for holding prisoners, in many places "prison quarters tended to be opportunistic, occupying structures."[5]

Regardless of the size of the confinement, what all prisons have in common is that they lead to social isolation and dependence. In this context, the consequences are less dramatic for people of higher social status who are punished for a short time than for people of lower social status who have to remain in confinement for an extended period of time. It is the personal resources and, of course, the willingness of relatives that could make imprisonment rather short-lived and bearable. There was the possibility to buy oneself out and thus influence imprisonment and its conditions. However, knowledge about the reasons for imprisonment and the chances of a trial was not open to every prisoner.

> Not much would have prevented a magistrate in a first-century Roman province from using the harsh conditions of imprisonment to alter an inmate's behavior, coerce a confession, settle a score, or hasten death—whether or not that inmate had been formally convicted.[6]

Ronald Grimes is *the* appropriate theorist to locate the everyday in the ritual not only because of his ritual approach but also because he has thoroughly studied ritual aspects in biblical texts. Fundamental to him is the speech act theory of J.L. Austin.

> Specifically, I will demonstrate the applicability of J.L. Austin's typology of "infelicitous" [his term] performances to both biblical and non-biblical examples of troublesome ritual. The reasons for putting speech act theory to this use are simple: (1) some of the examples used by Austin are ritualistic and (2) ritual contexts, more than any other, make use of what he calls performative utterance, that is, speech insofar as it accomplishes tasks rather than merely describing them.[7]

Grimes is concerned with speech act theory because rituals are expressed through language, and consequently, rituals can fail just as any other communicative act. "My hypothesis is that Austin's typology is applicable not only to things said in ritual contexts but also to things done in them, especially if the things done seem to go awry."[8] It is obvious to Grimes that the success of a ritual depends on the definition of ritual, and that it cannot be taken for granted that success or failure will be evaluated in the same way. But the question whether rituals must be fundamentally associated with emotions like, for example, happiness, success, truth, etc., or also reflect the opposites must be allowed. In the essay, Grimes proceeds by interrogating Austin's speech act theory on the question of unhappiness in ritual. Before we follow Grimes' argument further, we need to make a differentiation. I assume that rituals can succeed or fail regardless of the desired outcome. By this I mean that a ritual intended to bring about connectedness between meal participants can fail or succeed just as much as a ritual that marks social isolation. Any social, political, or religious evaluation can thus not be an integral part of the ritual performance. Grimes is not very precise at this point because the abovementioned speech act theory does not deal with the possible success of any ritual but is focused on the emotional consequence (here happy or infelicitous).[9]

Grimes is more aware of the limitations of the speech-act theory in other respects and adds two major aspects to the repertoire.

> "Glosses" are procedures that hide or ignore contradictions or major problems. Glossing over conflict is a function that rites proverbially (in anthropological theory) do well.
>
> In a "flop" all the procedures may be done correctly but the rite fails to resonate. It does not generate the proper tone, ethos, or atmosphere.[10]

For our search of ritual aspects in the so-called captivity letters, glossing provides us with an interesting observation. It can be assumed that in isolation and captivity hidden transcripts indeed play a role in different communication situations.[11] First, this is true for the distribution of messages via intermediaries and the scope of linguistic messages adapted to the possibilities and second for the choice of words that disguise the situation according to the circumstances. Third, and here the ritual framework becomes relevant, it applies to the thematization of rituals. In the description of ritual aspects, glossing can be done in very different ways. It is conceivable that the description of a successful ritual draws attention to realities just as much as the description of failure. In both cases, success or failure can turn out in favor of, or against, the detainee.

> I recently attended a wedding in which the bride was pregnant, followed a few months later by a child-blessing in which this same new wife participated with a black eye from her husband. Both ceremonies were "applied" in the same manner (and about as successfully) as her eye makeup. They "glossed" rather than "bridged" the chasms.[12]

The example of Grimes portrays very well that in this case the expectations toward a wedding are fully met. The bride or mother can only be miserably made up because violence in happy ritual settings does not correspond to the expectations of the ritual participants. In our situation, the rituals and the expectations associated with them are more complex because first it must be clarified whether the success or failure of a ritual in captivity is assumed.

2.2 *The Tension between Isolation and Community*

After setting out the theoretical framework and noting that rituals in captivity will be examined primarily for their everydayness and their capacity to gloss over realities, we will turn to the Pauline discourse and search for the meaning of isolation and community. We will only mention individual examples from the four captivity letters to sketch the discourse.

2.2.1 *The Lonely Captivity in the Letter to the Philippians*

The tension between isolation and community is evident in many places in Philippians, and especially in the opening. Being a "slave of Jesus Christ" (Phil 1:1) is charged with meaning for many exegetes.[13] John Gillman sees captivity located in the phrase alongside service to Christ. "This has a double nuance connoting both his identity as a servant of Christ as well as a captive of the Roman Empire."[14] Angela Standhartinger also considers an allusion to imprisonment possible, but points out that Paul is probably alone in captivity. Here, however, he speaks of himself and Timothy.[15] The following verses refer only to Paul, so that the tension between a solitary confinement and a confinement with a co-worker at the beginning of the letter is not resolved. Knowing this tension, Phil 1:7 adds another layer to the debate. Here, the Philippians are called his fellow-participants (συγκοινωνός). Indirectly, Timothy is replaced by the Philippians, for they share in his chains and in the gospel. Just as Timothy is a slave of Christ and of the Roman Empire with him, so are the Philippians. Phil 1:13 stands at the heart of Pauline theology, originally related to the captivity situation.

The decision about the evaluation of the socio-political background of the praetorium and about the grammatical reference of ἐν Χριστῷ ("in Christ") is above all crucial for our readiness to interpret the text metaphorically or in a figurative sense. In this respect, the praetorium can be taken not only for a building but also for a group of people, the guard. The grammatical reference ἐν Χριστῷ is preferably translated as referring to φανερός γενέσθαι ("to become known"). In this, Christ is the cause of the bonds, and he acts through and in captivity. Standhartinger translates "so that my chains have been made manifest in Christ." This interpretation puts a different emphasis on the theology of the body since it is not Christ but the chains that are made manifest in the captivity. Consequently, Christ does not act through suffering or in an agonizing situation that brings body and mind to their limits.[16] It is convincing at this point to understand Pauline Christology not as anti-body. Especially because the proclamation of the gospel requires courage and does not stand in the way of its dissemination (Phil 1:14). Phil 1:21 confirms the impression that Paul attaches theological relevance to isolation: Paul affirms that living, for him, is Christ and dying is gain—a constellation that could only be validated for him in captivity. As if there had not been this convincing presentation of the captivity situation, Paul alludes to entirely different ways of proclaiming it. Paul wants to leave, and he seems to be able to decide whether to remain in isolation or to rejoin the community (Phil 1:22–24). This juxtaposition is mirrored in these verses by another extreme—suicide. If one sees his suicide as an expression of one's own will in isolation, then this corresponds both to the possibilities within imprisonment and to a theological self-understanding according to which Paul, and like him any believer, has the innate power to decide for Christ, that is, for life.[17] In the rest of the letter, Paul establishes images of community.

> Ministering to Paul, and evidently bolstering his spirit, is Epaphroditus, Paul's brother, coworker, fellow soldier, and messenger from the

community (Phil 2:25–30). It is unknown whether this coworker lived with Paul in prison or was arrested when he brought money from the Philippians to support Paul.

(Phil 4:18)[18]

Furthermore, at the end of the letter, Paul considers himself a great influencer, since he includes the whole house of the emperor in his proclamation (Phil 4:22). Thus, the letter ends as it began: with an imperial claim from captivity. The letter to the Philippians describes a solitary imprisonment that is nevertheless closely linked to the political context and the associated metaphors.

2.2.2 *No Tension in the Letter to the Colossians*

In the letter to the Colossians, the tension is comparatively weak. We will discuss the ritual references in the following section and find them to be more expressive than in the letter to the Philippians. At this point, it should only be pointed out that the ritual variety is in favor of the community. The letter to the Colossians presents a different picture of tensions between isolation and community. Its focus is on communal aspects. This becomes most evident in Col 1:24, where Paul assumes that he suffers and rejoices for the sake of the community. At the end of the letter, he asks the readers to remember his bonds. In this, we observe the attempt to depict captivity as rather positive, with little reference to harsh conditions (Col 4:18). Standhartinger correctly assesses that the letter to the Colossians paints a picture of an apostle surrounded only by the closest intimates (Col 4:10–5).

Here, imprisonment has already become a metaphor of death (Col 4:2–3), and the apostolic suffering receives soteriological quality (Col 1:24–25).[19] Another indication of the metaphorization of isolation is the use of the term "slave" in Colossians. The much-discussed statement that slaves should remain with their worldly masters must not go unmentioned in this context. The exhortation is so clearly non-metaphorical that the discrepancy between the possible metaphorical expressions about Paul, the slave of Christ, is addressed. It is understandable that in Colossians, Paul addresses worldly slaves in his community and urges them to remain in their position. In the history of post-colonial research, it is disputed whether this state of bondage can actually be understood as an expression of their service to Christ. However, we can focus on the fact that the letter to the Colossians does not only establish tensions between the metaphorical and the non-metaphorical, but also distinctions between forms of isolation and domination by a third party. On the one hand, foreign domination by worldly masters is established for the service of Christ, and on the other hand, captivity through philosophy and empty promises is urged. Paul criticizes intellectual and cultic captivity in Col 2:8. "See to it that no one takes you captive through philosophy and empty deceit, according to human tradition, according to the elemental spirits of the universe, and not according to Christ." Human traditions and worldly elements, according to Paul, do not correspond to Christ. This example has shown that it is noteworthy that human traditions are associated with philosophy and empty deceit, but immediate imprisonment in dungeons and chains is portrayed more positively by metaphorization.

2.2.3 *The Inversion of the Hierarchical System in the Letter to Philemon*

In Colossians, we have seen how Paul relates the terms "imprisonment" and "isolation" to intellectual aspects and thus distracts from his immediate social distance, which is further reinforced by the metaphorization of the chains. In the Epistle to Philemon, Pauline theology around isolation and community is turned upside down. Gillman concludes:

> Ironically, the imprisoned Paul has inverted the hierarchical system. He has become the father to the slave master Philemon, having brought him into the faith (Phlm 1:19), as he has become the father to his adopted son Onesimus (Phlm 1:10). By expecting Philemon to accept Onesimus back as a brother, Paul gives them the same status, thus transforming the master-slave power dynamic into a relationship of equals in the ekklesia.[20]

Again, Paul, the prisoner of Christ, writes from captivity and distracts from a situation of his own by raising his voice and interceding on behalf of the slave Onesimus. Furthermore, the letter is focused on community. Apart from the close associates who link this letter to Colossians (Col 4:10–14; Phlm 1:23–24), the letter is addressed to the sister Aphia and Archippus, the fellow combatant, indeed the whole community in Philemon's house (Phlm 1:2).

2.2.4 *The Social Status and Imprisonment in the Letter to the Ephesians*

In the letter to the Ephesians, imprisonment is not only addressed between the lines, so that there is a striking closeness to the other letters.[21]

> Here he commands slaves to be obedient to their earthly masters (Eph 6:5; see Col 3:22). But Paul doesn't stop there. He elevates their status, calling them "slaves of Christ." Paul goes one step further, admonishing them to do "the will of God from the heart" and to serve with enthusiasm the Lord (literally Master) and not human beings (Eph 6:6–7). Although Paul does not call for an end to slavery, this principle is nothing less than subversive.[22]

Eph 6:5, 6–7, and Eph 6:9 testify that the bond between masters and slaves is above their separation based on status. Respect on the one hand, but above all the common position under the authority of God provide for an immanent community. This is contradicted only by Eph 3:1; 4:1; 6:20. In these verses, Paul speaks of "his bonds." Paul characterizes himself as a prisoner, but a prisoner "for Jesus Christ" or "in the Lord."

2.3 *Personal and Collective Experiences of Crisis*

Having investigated the tension between isolation and community in the captivity letters, we now turn to the ritual content of the letters. We explore the question of which ritual practices are included in the letters and how they relate to the tension between isolation and community.

The ritual world of the captivity letters is dominated by prayer language. Prayers and talking about prayers are generally very common in the New Testament writings. Well known are especially the hymns and traditional prayers based on oral sources. However, the meanings of prayers in the biblical narratives are also examined. In other contexts, it could be shown that Luke, for example, connects meal reports with the topos of prayer at various places in his narrative and repeatedly interweaves Peter into the plot. In addition, through the theme of discipleship, prayer connects the believers with God on the vertical level and with each other on the horizontal level. The place where this takes place is, among other things, the common meal. Ritual aspects are used in the Gospel to set theological emphases. In Luke's Gospel it is, among other things, the community meal which is also structurally embedded in the Gospel. These emphases are on discipleship and community. In the captivity letters, the emphasis is on isolation. It is advisable, for the consideration of prayers in the New Testament, to examine the different terms that can be perceived as prayer language. The verb εὐχαριστέω ("to be grateful, to give thanks") is generally regarded as a key term to refer to a prayer practice. This verb is further defined in Greek by prefixes. In New Testament writings, and specifically in the captivity letters, we find variants such as προσεύχομαι, since it can also be understood as praying as such; the prefix conveys the aspect of actively turning in prayer. The semantic field also includes the term δέησις that refers to a request. (The German equivalent would be "Bittgebet.") Theologically very complex is also εὐχαριστία. In contrast to a complex reception history, the meanings of the occurrences in the New Testament can be summarized as "gratitude" and "thanksgiving." Of course, the semantic field of prayer also includes places or ritual settings that contain prayers. Baptism, meal fellowship, and the life of associations play an important role here. On this basis, we will now look at the semantic field of the ritual world of the captivity letters. The following overview will show that these elements were taken up from different sides.[23]

The letter to the Philippians uses the following semantic field. The variants εὐχαριστέω ("to be grateful, to give thanks," Phil 1:3), προσεύχομαι ("to pray," Phil 1:9), and εὐχαριστία ("gratitude", "thanksgiving," Phil 4:6) are noteworthy compared to the other letters. No other letter uses all three terms. In addition, no other letter uses the term δέησις as frequently (Phil 1:4, 19). It connotes a request for a specific thing or help and is not only a mere prayer. In Phil 1:4, the focus on the matter is clearly visible because prayer becomes matter. Paul speaks of his active role as a prayer warrior by combining δέησις with ποιέω ("to make"). In Phil 1:19, the request is σωτηρία ("salvation"), though prayer is not the only reason for σωτηρία since the Spirit of Jesus Christ also provides it. Phil 4:6 summarizes very well the importance of prayer for the letter. Here, in terms of history of tradition, we can perceive references both to the Jesus prayer practice (Q) and to the prayer tradition of Psalms. Not only δέησις and εὐχαριστία but also αἴτημα ("request," Phil 4:6) point to a tension between personal concerns and formal petitions. The appropriateness of prayer language to convey messages about oneself and a captivity situation has already been proven on the example of the Philippians hymn. If, as indicated above, the possibility of the apostle's solitary confinement is also debated, then the references to the "hidden transcripts" in prayer language support this tendency. Not worrying about anything and facing God in prayer points to prayers and petitions that do address God immediately despite a relatively self-determined starting point. In keeping with the image of the apostle alone, leading the community, the prayer language shows no evidence of a communal ritual.

Prayer language is also present in Colossians, but less varied than in Philippians. Giving thanks and praying are directly related to each other in Col 1:3. In Col 1:9, this mutual reinforcement is taken up, but not expressed with εὐχαριστέω and προσεύχομαι, but with προσεύχομαι and αἰτέω ("to ask, request"). Intercession becomes more specific when Col 1:12 states that thanksgiving should be expressed "with joy" (μετὰ χαρᾶς). The result of this joy is described shortly thereafter in Col 2:12 as εὐχαριστία and then moves into more complex ritual worlds.

Col 2:11–12 and Col 2:16–17 even go so far as to embellish customary ritual practices: "In him also you were circumcised with a spiritual circumcision, by putting off the body of the flesh in the circumcision of Christ; when you were buried with him in baptism, you were also raised with him through faith in the power of God, who raised him from the dead" (Col 2:11–12). The juxtaposition of spiritual circumcision versus carnal circumcision is not very accurate. The word ἀπέκδυσις ("removal") expresses that a circumcision, which is carried out by hand, is to be contrasted with the circumcision of Jesus Christ. The genitive in the words ἐν τῇ περιτομῇ τοῦ Χριστοῦ ("in the circumcision of Christ") can refer not only to circumcision of the body of Jesus or mean circumcision in the manner of Jesus but can also refer to the means. Following this thought, more context needs to be considered by investigating how the circumcision is carried out: by the hands (ἐν τῇ ἀπεκδύσει) or by Jesus Christ (ἐν τῇ περιτομῇ τοῦ Χριστοῦ). Further ritual practices (Col 2:12) commence with entombment and baptism leading to the raising (of the dead). In these verses, the letter to the Colossians traces a ritual consequence which, strikingly, does not go into details but, of course, gives a direction.

"Therefore do not let anyone condemn you in matters of food and drink or of observing festivals, new moons, or sabbaths. These are only a shadow of what is to come, but the substance belongs to Christ" (Col 2:16–17). Food and drink are placed in a trans-regional, trans-denominational, and trans-social context in these verses. What is also important here is not the knowledge about eating and drinking at a certain festival at a certain time. What is important is that ritual competence shall not be questioned when it comes to the ritual performance. Chapters 3 and 4 remain theologically oriented in the best sense and thrive on the community as calls to thanksgiving and prayer. In the tension between isolation and community, it is noticeable that Paul expresses himself critically toward the actions of man. Human traditions are only conditionally compatible with Christ, which is also evident in ritual action.

In the letter to Philemon, the ritual sphere is very reduced and cannot serve as a contact space between Paul and the outside world. Also, prayer language would not be the means of choice to change hierarchies. To thank God in prayer is a phrase that is not further elaborated during the letter and also does not come into play in δέησις ("request," Phil 4:6).

The letter to the Ephesians presents a balanced picture of prayer language and ritual actions that play a role in the context of the text. In the previous section, we have observed a focus on Paul as a person acting with the authority of God in the community. Eph 1:16 confirms this impression by using εὐχαριστέω ("to be grateful, to give thanks"). Paul prays for others in his prayers. This segues into imitation or exemplary behavior, which is used as an occasion in Chapter 5 to avoid all other forms of ritual performance apart from giving thanks. In Eph 6:18, this picture of the apostle is confirmed with προσεύχομαι, δέησις. By analogy with Col 4:2–4, Paul repeats his call to the community. They are not to cease from prayer. The call to prayer is repeated, but not to corporate prayer or any other ritual action. The reference to Paul succeeds only through the intercession of the community for Paul, which he also claims for himself in these verses.

3 Conclusion

Examining the captivity letters collectively and regardless of authorship indeed has a long tradition within New Testament scholarship. Studies on the socio-historical specifics of captivity conditions in early Christianity have contributed to thinking about hidden transcripts in these letters. The "hidden transcripts" are an essential part in various communication situations that can bridge isolation or reconcile conflicts of interest. In prayer language, communication situations overlap as needs and interests are expressed and negotiated. If a prayer is placed in a captive situation in a ritual context, then understanding the "hidden transcripts" becomes a social skill. I have followed this lead and perceived the Pauline discourse in its entirety on the topic. On different levels, the letters have shown how social isolation is dealt with on the one hand. Ritual language and the enactment of ritual practices have been examined for their relationship to the tension between isolation and community. A surprising result of this examination is that the dominant prayer language did not resolve the tension. Competing with dealing with immanent or constructed experiences of confinement and isolation, the ritual aspects conveyed through the letters support these accounts. It has become obvious that where isolation is not resolved, ritual does not compensate for it either. Consequently, ritual aspects of writing do not only serve to build community but can also stabilize the opposite, namely isolation. Subsequent studies will have to investigate whether social isolation, including metaphorical social isolation, and experiences of distance are best dealt with when cultural ritual experiences make this exceptional situation bearable.

Notes

1 Standhartinger, "Welt," 140–141.
2 Al-Suadi, "Ritual Experience," 104.
3 Grimes, "Typen," 120, 123.
4 Grimes, "Typen," 123.
5 Skinner, "Remember," 270.
6 Skinner, "Remember," 272.
7 Grimes, "Performances," 104.
8 Grimes, "Performances," 104.
9 Grimes, "Performances," 106: He employs a set of classifications that (1) enable us to distinguish words that say something ("constatives") from those that do something ("performatives"), and (2) help us judge when performatives are "happy," on the one hand, or "infelicitous," on the other. Here I am concerned with types of "infelicitous performance" and the light they shed on failed ritual.
10 Grimes, "Performances," 112, 113.
11 Laura Robinson is discussing counter-imperial or anti-imperial interpretations of the New Testament, which she defines as a reading that looks for allusions or hidden meanings expressing dissatisfaction with Rome. Robinson, "Hidden," 57; note 5.
12 Grimes, "Performances," 112.
13 A metaphorical interpretation is proposed, for example, by Annette Merz: "Paul refers to himself (and his co-workers) as a 'slave of Christ' (δοῦλος Χριστοῦ) in Rom 1:1, Gal 1:10, and Phil 1:1. In 1 Cor 7:22, the metaphor describes any free person who responded to the 'call' (I will use this Pauline expression throughout the present article) and became a believer." Merz, "Believers," 100.
14 Gillman, "Voice," 347.
15 Standhartinger, *Philipperbrief*, 73.
16 Standhartinger, *Philipperbrief*, 98–104.
17 Gillman, "Voice," 347.
18 Gillman, "Voice," 348.
19 Standhartinger, "Welt," 140–141.
20 Gillman, "Voice," 351.
21 Gillman, "Voice," 352: Paul states three times that he is "in chains" (Eph 3:1; 4:1; 6:20). Like in the other letters, he is a prisoner "for Christ Jesus" (Eph 3:1) and "in the Lord" (Eph 4:1).
22 Gillman, "Voice," 352.
23 Al-Suadi, "Petrus," 540.

Bibliography

Al-Suadi, Soham, "Petrus im Spiegel des Antiochenischen Konflikts im Lukanischen Doppelwerk," *Theologische Zeitschrift* 4, no. 69 (2013): 24–52.

Al-Suadi, Soham, "Ritual Experience and Emotions: The Right Place for Water Rites in Luke-Acts," in *The Ritual World of Ancient Christianity: Rites, Emotions, Identities*, edited by Soham Al-Suadi, Richard S. Ascough, and DeMaris, Richard. London: Routledge, 2021, 103–117.
Gillman, John, "Paul's Voice Still Resounds in His Letters from Prison," *Word & World* 38, no. 4 (2018): 345–354.
Grimes, Ronald L., "Infelicitious Performances and Ritual Criticism," *Semeia* 41 (1988): 103–122.
Grimes, Ronald L., "Typen ritueller Erfahrung," in *Ritualtheorien*, edited by Andréa Belliger, Stuttgart: Springer, 2013, 119–134.
Merz, Annette, "Believers as 'Slaves of Christ' and 'Freed Persons of the Lord': Slavery and Freedom as Ambiguous Soteriological Metaphors in 1 Cor 7:22 and Col 3:22–4:1," *Journal for Theology and the Study of Religion* 72, no. 2 (2018): 95–110.
Robinson, Laura, "Hidden Transcripts? The Supposedly Self-Censoring Paul and Rome as Surveillance State in Modern Pauline Scholarship," *New Testament Studies* 67, no. 1 (2021): 55–72.
Skinner, Matthew L., "Remember My Chains: New Testament Perspectives on Incarceration," *Interpretation* 72, no. 3 (2018): 269–281.
Standhartinger, Angela, "Aus der Welt eines Gefangenen: Die Kommunikationsstruktur des Philipperbriefs im Spiegel seiner Abfassungssituation," *Novum Testamentum* 55, no. 2 (2013): 140–167.
Standhartinger, Angela, *Der Philipperbrief* (Handbuch zum Neuen Testament 11/1), Tübingen: Mohr Siebeck, 2021.

Part III

Plagues, Infections, and Witchcraft

9 Plagues, Withdrawal, and Wayfaring in the Hebrew Bible[1]

Elisa Uusimäki

1 Introduction

The story of the ten plagues that struck the Egyptians because the Pharaoh refused to free the Hebrews continues to live on in the Western imagination, from music to visual arts to cinema. Many people recognize references to the exodus story (Exod 7:1–12:31), regardless of their general level of biblical literacy, because of its catchy details and powerful replications in art and entertainment. Yet the Hebrew Bible tells us more about ancient perceptions of plagues than this famous tale of liberation. In this article, I analyze literary and cultural representations of plagues in the Hebrew Bible with a focus on the theme of movement.[2] By exploring links between plagues and (im)mobility, I draw attention to imaginations of and responses to health crises in the ancient eastern Mediterranean world.

The question of plagues and (im)mobility is timely as COVID-19 has urged virtually any person around the globe to consider their relation to movement. During the pandemic, there have been travel bans and border closures, which have affected both travelers and their hosts. However, the effects of COVID-19 on human mobility have not been limited to long-distance or regional travel but have been felt in daily life along with various civil restrictions and recommendations to practice social distancing. Those affected by the virus and their near contacts have also been subject to isolation and quarantine procedures. These actions have helped to limit the spread of the virus, but they have come at a cost, including social disruptions and issues of mental health.[3] This article examines texts in the the Hebrew Bible which point to how things slow down during plagues. Yet, some biblical narratives suggest the opposite: at times, plagues may increase movement when a chaotic situation shakes the status quo and enables an otherwise unimaginable relocation.

There are a handful of related terms in Biblical Hebrew which simply get translated into the one English word "plague." The most common one of them is נגע (*nega'*), but the terms דבר (*dever*), מגפה (*maggefah*), מכה (*makkah*), נגף (*negef*), קטב (*qetev*), and רשף (*reshef*) also refer to miscellaneous pestilences.[4] They are often presented as part of a wider cosmic plan, as punishments through which YHWH, the God of Israel, shows his majesty and

DOI: 10.4324/b22930-12

power over life and death.[5] They also serve as threats, warning the Hebrews not to ignore divine requests.[6] Meanwhile, there are texts that do not speculate on the cause or purpose of such harms but point to practical management strategies, thus indicating preparation for and resilience during difficult times. For example, people may visit a sanctuary to offer sacrifices or pray to avoid or free themselves from plagues.[7] Some texts, in turn, promote quarantine as a means of managing infectious disease (see more below).[8]

While the Hebrew Bible shows some concern for health-related issues, one needs to keep in mind that it is a collection of writings put together for a religious purpose, here mainly to serve as scripture. The texts were not written or compiled to illuminate or record practices of daily life in ancient Israel. Furthermore, the perspective provided by the text's final form is that of scribal elites who edited it to reflect their own agendas and worldviews. As such, the corpus does not express the views of all Israelites and Judeans/Jews. Yet, a close reading of it may reveal conceptions of healthcare as the ancient authors understood them.[9]

In what follows, I investigate notions of plagues in the Hebrew Bible with a focus on how they are imagined to either prompt people to move or hinder them from doing so. I begin with analyzing the representation of plagues as a catalyst for liberation in two narratives; these tales draw attention to how YHWH, here depicted in the role of a divine puppet master, uses them to control things. I then examine the evidence of legal, narrative, and poetic texts describing isolation caused by illness, which is characterized by the plague idiom and thus presumed to be infectious. While biblical laws concentrate on how to handle a plague, poetic literature elaborates on how it feels to be hit by one.

2 Plagues Prompting Mobility

While plagues are harmful, the misfortune of one group can help or even save another. This dynamic is illustrated by two narratives, in which plagues cause welcome disruptions, enabling the release of the Hebrews who find themselves stuck in undesirable situations.

Genesis, to begin with, contains mythical tales of ancient patriarchs and their families, including one about the time of Sarai and Abram (later known as Sarah and Abraham) in Egypt. The couple is said to have moved there owing to a famine (Gen 12:10).[10] The story is narrated from the viewpoint of Abram, who is anxious that Egyptians might kill him because of his wife's beauty, asking Sarai to present herself as his sister (12:13).[11] The locals indeed recognize the beauty of Sarai who is taken to the Pharaoh's palace (12:14–15). The ruler treats Abram well because of having acquired Sarai, giving him slaves and animals in exchange (12:16). However, YHWH expresses his discontent with the situation by causing perilous harm, afflicting the Pharaoh's household with "mighty plagues" (נגעים גדלים, *nega'im gedolim*) (12:17).[12] The angry ruler then sends Abram away with his wife and possessions (12:18–20).

In this tale of economic migration, Sarai and Abram leave Canaan in the hope of better material prospects. Abram's plot to take advantage of Sarai's attractiveness to improve his own prospects in a precarious situation follows a pattern known from several societies: the migrant woman is exposed to a type of sex work with the purpose of guaranteeing the family's financial success.[13] Yet the outcome, Sarai's placement in the foreign palace, results in the partners' separation. A God-sent plague solves the tricky situation by prompting the Pharaoh, horrified by the raging plague, to deport the couple from his country. This event of forced mobility serves as an act of deliverance. Having benefited from his deceptive deal, Abram leaves Egypt with wealth, embarking on a journey back to the land promised to him by YHWH earlier in the narrative (13:1–4).

The patriarchal narratives involve many incidents of mobility, including but not limited to the story of Sarai and Abram in Egypt.[14] Yet this tale is relevant to the wider Pentateuchal narrative since it contains the first reference to Egypt in Genesis and prefigures the ambiguity that characterizes the relation between Israel and Egypt later on. For Israel, Egypt is a place of both shelter and mortal danger.[15] The patriarchal narratives are followed by the Joseph novella (Gen 37–50), which explains how the Hebrews ended up thriving in Egypt. Their circumstances in the new country of residence deteriorate, however, and the following exodus story is another tale in which plagues caused by divine intervention serve to deliver Hebrews who find themselves in an oppressive situation in a foreign land.[16]

The plot begins to unfold as Moses and Aaron consult the Pharaoh about the possibility to offer a sacrifice in the wilderness to avoid YHWH hitting the Hebrews with a plague (דבר, *dever*; Exod 5:3). The Pharaoh does not consent to the request, accusing the Hebrews of laziness (5:4–5). YHWH encourages Moses to continue the negotiation process (6:1–13, 28–30; 7:1–13) and eventually decides to discipline the Egyptians to free the Hebrews. This happens through a series of ten cosmic terrors, which increase gradually in severity, including an act of turning water into blood, frogs, vermin, swarms of insects, rinderpest, boils, hail, locusts, darkness, and the death of the first-born (7:14–12:36).[17] The terrors are coercive as well as demonstrating the power of YHWH, who defeats the Egyptian deities.[18]

Yet the Pharaoh refuses to permit the departure. Only the final terror and the subsequent lament throughout the Egyptian households terrify him to the extent that he urges the Hebrews to leave the country (12:30–36, esp. 12:33). The night of horror and chaos caused by the tenth terror is fundamental to the cultural memory and cultic calendar of the Jewish tradition as it installs the celebration of the Passover festival (12:1–28); the collective memory of the terrors in Egypt also lingers on in other biblical stories and poetry.[19]

It is customary to refer to the ten terrors as ten plagues, but the term "plague" (נגע, *nega'*) first appears in Exod 11:1, when YHWH announces the last plague to Moses, while it is not used of the nine terrors depicted in Exod 7–10. In fact, not all of them are plagues in the medical sense of the word.

Most of them are typical, albeit exaggerated, natural phenomena. Yet the fifth (rinderpest, דבר, *dever*), sixth (boils, שחין, *shekhin*; אבעבעת, *'ava'bu'ot*), and tenth (the death of the first-borns, מת כל-בקר, *met kol-bekor*) terrors seem to involve infectious diseases, posing a direct danger for the health and life of humans and/or animals.[20] This is obvious regarding rinderpest and boils (9:1–12) but also seems to apply to the tenth terror, the death of the first-borns, for the Hebrews must undertake ritual procedures and withdraw to their homes to avoid the death of their own first-born when YHWH passes through to strike the Egyptians (12:21–28). A link to plagues is established by the Hebrew root used of "striking" (נגף, *n-g-p*), since it also underlines the term נגף (*negef*), "plague."

In Genesis 12, YHWH is imagined as a liberator of his people who controls illness and may cause even mortal harm to those who hurt the Hebrews. While the ten terrors harm the Egyptian "other," the wider exodus story connects plagues with the Hebrews. As the thirsty and tired people complain about the harsh conditions in the wilderness upon their departure from Egypt, YHWH motivates them by promising not to send a plague as long as his commandments are kept (Exod 15:26, cf. Num 14:11–12). Yet the people break the covenant by building a golden calf, which prompts YHWH to strike them with a plague (Exod 32:35). YHWH also punishes the Hebrews with plagues later during the wilderness wandering, owing to their greed, rebellion, and idolatry.[21] Plagues thus serve as instruments of divine justice that may strike YHWH's own people, whether for cultic or ethical reasons.

In summary, plagues are mentioned in two Hebrew Bible narratives as a means to set people free: it is after a plague that Sarai and Abram exit from Egypt where they had stayed as economic migrants, and after yet another plague, God delivers the Hebrews, this time as a collective, from Egypt. While plagues signal divine help in undesirable situations, they also harm the Hebrews as a divine punishment, and the authors invoke their threat to urge obedience and compliance. These texts on the mythical past do not help us to reconstruct historical events, but they point to a conviction of YHWH's power over maladies. They imply a moody deity who uses biological weapons to help his people but does not shy away from punishing them by the same means in case of unpleasing conduct.

3 Plagues, Isolation, and Immobility

While plagues cause welcome disruptions in some narratives, they are undesirable to those hurt by them and may sometimes hinder movement instead of permitting it. Various biblical texts also reveal and reflect on this side of the coin. I will next investigate priestly laws and narratives suggesting that a person affected by a plague should withdraw and isolate themselves. I then analyze liturgical poetry on human experiences of loneliness and longing caused by illness-related seclusion. In these texts, plague imagery is frequently used to describe illness, which suggests that these illnesses are considered infectious, and isolation is prompted by a desire to avoid further spread of the plague or to calm down an already raging one.

The Hebrew Bible mentions "healing" (רפא, *r-p-'*), that is, restoration and recovery, but does not contain detailed information on medical techniques.[22] Instead, the authors stress YHWH's role as the one who both causes illness and cures (e.g., Exod 15:26; Job 5:18). Yet humans, too, feature as health care personnel. Prophets are depicted as legitimate healers (e.g., 2 Kgs 4, 5, 8; 2 Kgs 20), whereas priests are assigned to serve in the process of identifying and managing illness.[23] A modern distinction between the "religious" and the "medical" realm does not apply; therefore, questions of healthcare appear as "cultural products" tied to ideological and religious views.[24]

In Leviticus, laws presented as divine revelation delivered to Moses and Aaron provide us with an ideological take on the priests' job description. They are known for their sacrificial duties and administration of the sanctuary but also serve as health care consultants. It has been argued that a priest is not primarily a healer but a sort of inspector.[25] Yet he prescribes a combination of rituals and medical procedures. To protect the community from the threat of disease, the task of a priest, characterized as "the purificatory priest" (הכהן המטהר, *hakohen hametaher*) in Lev 14:11, is to prescribe measures that may involve sacrifices, ritual washing, or quarantine. Their purpose is to purify those whose physical conditions are regarded as unclean owing to some cause of impurity (טמאה, *tum'ah*).[26] In priestly thinking, impurity is regarded as preventing one from participating in the cult, and its removal is needed to achieve an ideal state of purity that enables one to be in the presence of the deity and join the public worship.[27]

Purification processes are compiled in Lev 12–15 with laws on the mother and her newborn child (ch. 12), contagious skin ailments (ch. 13–14), and infectious discharges linked with genital organs (ch. 15).[28] For us, it is relevant that the section in Lev 13:1–46 discusses acute cases of skin ailment in human beings as well as related measures of diagnosis, while Lev 14:1–32 outlines purification rites needed to remove the impurity caused by skin ailment.[29] Ch. 13 begins with the following statement, which introduces the key term "scaly infection" (13:2):

> When a person has on the skin of their body a swelling, a rash, or a discoloration, and it develops into a scaly infection (לנגע צרעת, *lenega' tsara'at*) on the skin of their body, it shall be reported to Aaron the priest or to one of his sons, the priests.

The term used for "scaly infection" consists of two words, נגע (*nega'*) and צרעת (*tsara'at*).[30] Though *tsara'at* is often translated as "leprosy," it does not denote the modern disease known by that name.[31] Instead, *tsara'at* is a collective medical term referring to several skin ailments.[32] It is never classified as a "defect" (מאום, *m'um*) in the Hebrew Bible, but those affected by this somatic condition are marginalized just as those suffering from various defects.[33] Here, *tsara'at* is combined with נגע (*nega'*, "plague" or "affection"), which frequently refers, together with other derivatives of the root נגע (*n-g-'*), to an affection, affected person, or affected articles in Lev 13.[34] Since the term connotes a plague and the following verses elaborate on quarantine practices, the text can be said to concern immobility associated with a type of "plague."

Lev 13 outlines several cases of inspecting *tsara'at*, but I focus here on the issue of withdrawal in the light of the first section on symptomatology (13:1–8).[35] As quoted, a person exhibiting symptoms is to be taken to a priest (13:2) for examination as to whether he or she suffers from an acute skin ailment. There are different possible outcomes (13:3–8). Clear symptoms – a white discoloration of the body hair and lesions deeper than the surrounding skin – lead to proclaiming the person impure (טמא, *t-m-'*).[36] The lack of obvious symptoms means that the possibly affected person is held for further examination. He or she is confined (הסגיר, *hisgir*) for seven days, only to undergo another inspection.[37] If the symptoms have not worsened, another seven-day quarantine takes place. Then the person is pronounced pure (טהר, *t-h-r*), given that the affection has faded. Yet, if the rash spreads on the skin thereafter, the person is declared impure indefinitely because of *tsara'at*.

Even minor symptoms should thus result in withdrawal, which ensures that the potentially ill person does not infect others in the community and render them incapable of taking part in public worship. However, the text does not specify the particularities of the procedure. Another law in the same chapter (13:46) simply states that a person continues to be impure as long as he or she is affected and should live "alone" (בדד, *badad*) and "outside the camp" (מחוץ למחנה, *mikhuts lamakhaneh*) (cf. Num 5:2; 12:14–15). This omission may pertain to the fact that Leviticus describes a utopian community instead of a real one.[38] Its laws were composed by priestly elites and were probably never enforced across all of society. Instead, they portray *ideals*, including the aesthetic norm of spotless skin.[39] The emphatic concern of the laws for collective purity may pertain to the processing of the trauma of loss that followed Jerusalem's destruction and the Babylonian exile in the 6th century BCE.[40]

While it is unclear to what extent social isolation owing to skin ailments was practiced in ancient Israel, the priestly elite thought about and acknowledged the need for quarantine. Furthermore, the regulations were presumably subject to some dissemination among laypeople, who are the implied audience of Leviticus.[41] Yet, even if some people implemented the procedure outlined in Leviticus, this hardly applied to all members of the society; for example, the impracticalities of confinement for women taking care of young children or for someone living in an agrarian community and needing to work with others to support themselves and their families would have been immense.

Even if the priestly laws cannot be taken at face value as if they represented daily customs, there is some further evidence to support the prospect of social isolation and quarantine practices in ancient Israel. First, the Mesopotamian material suggests that people with skin conditions were expelled from the city and excluded from society.[42] Similarly, 2 Kings 7:3 mentions four men with a skin disease (מצרעים, *metsora'im*) who sit outside the gate of Samaria. While the passing reference leaves many questions unanswered, it suggests that people with infectious diseases could be excluded from the rest of the society and left at the city gate "to beg or to perform undesirable tasks" to survive.[43] Such exclusion would turn ill people into forced migrants and internally displaced outcasts in their homelands.

Second, two parallel stories in the Hebrew Bible suggest that elites suffering from *tsara'at* had the privilege to isolate. They concern a king of Judah (8th c. BCE) called Azariah in the Deuteronomistic history and Uzziah in the Chronicles. According to both versions, YHWH strikes the king, owing to his cultic sins, with a skin ailment that bothers him until his death (2 Kgs 15:1–7; 2 Chr 26:16–21).[44] Both texts also mention that the king lived "in a separate house" (2 Kgs 15:5; 2 Chr 26:21), which implies an infectious disease posing a threat to others.[45] Meanwhile, the story about Naaman in 2 Kings 5:1–15 contradicts such a practice. This commander of the king of Aram (9th c. BCE) suffers from a skin ailment (מצרע, *metsora'*) and embarks on a journey after his wife's slave girl tells him about a prophet-healer in Samaria. Israel's king is suspicious of the foreigner, but Elisha urges a healing process. In this tale, the entrance of an impure person into Israelite society is not restricted, which shows that the biblical responses to infectious illness are not consistent.

Priestly laws portray ideal social realities, therefore, while some narratives depict elites isolating during illness. In both cases, they do not deal with average persons in society and should not be considered as the basis of common social practices in antiquity. They nevertheless suggest that quarantine could be undertaken by those who took priestly regulations seriously and/or could afford it. In addition, the passing reference in 2 Kings 7:3 exhibits the marginalized position of those excluded from society because of carrying infectious diseases. The psalms add to this picture by including expressions of seclusion. They highlight that illness is never just about the body but involves mental and social aspects as well.

Though ancient poetic texts such as psalms do not offer immediate insights into anyone's inner life, they are not fully detached from lived experiences. Remaining public representations of the self, poetic texts point to something beyond such a construction, for example, "aspects of the individuality, subjectivity, and uniqueness of the particular persons behind the voices."[46] Given the frequent use of the first-person voice, psalms also invite new audiences to share and take part in the speaker's sentiment, which points to the text as a sort of archive of stereotypical experiences across time and place.[47]

Several psalms express wishes to communicate with the deity at times of trouble (e.g., Pss 22:2–3; 88:2–3, 14–15), and some of them refer to illness and healing in particular.[48] In a few cases, the speaker uses the term "plague" to describe his or her illness. The plea to YHWH in Ps 39:11 is a case in point: "Take away your plague (נגעך, *nig'ekha*) from me; I perish from your blows." The lament of Psalm 38, one of the seven penitential psalms in the later Christian tradition, is another illuminating example.[49] The speaker recounts his or her encounter with illness, interpreting it as a punishment for sins and turning to YHWH on whom his or her misery and prospective healing depend (38:1–5). After the initial lament and appeal, the speaker details his or her bodily experience (38:6–13):

> My wounds stink and rot because of my folly. I am all bent and bowed; I walk about in gloom all day long. For my sinews are full of fever; there is no soundness in my flesh. I am all benumbed and crushed; I roar because of the turmoil in my heart. O YHWH, you are aware of all my longings; my sighing is not hidden from you. My heart palpitates; my strength has left me; the light of my eyes – I have lost it, as well. My friends and companions stand back from my plague (נגעי, *nig'i*); my neighbours stand far off. Those who seek my life lay traps; those who wish me harm speak malice; they utter deceit all the time.

The vivid description highlights the physical pain and discomfort of illness, including the decay or even loss of certain physiological functions, as well as associated psychological and social consequences.[50] The speaker feels alienated from his or her close ones who keep away from him or her because of the "plague." The mention of such distance reveals a feeling of being shunned by close ones because of illness; malady thus highlights the disparity between people, disrupts social relations, and causes feelings of solitude.[51]

In sum, biblical responses to plagues involve immobility. The authors of priestly laws and some narratives are aware of related health risks and mention or endorse exclusion and quarantine practices.[52] Liturgical poems draw attention to physical and mental well-being during illness by elaborating on experiences of pain, loneliness, and longing.

4 Conclusion

For many of us today, COVID-19 has been the first personal experience of a pandemic. Related anxieties are something we share with one another around the globe, but aspects of the experience also tie us with those who lived before us. In ancient Israel, too, plagues prompted both affective experiences and practical responses. In the ideal world of biblical texts, just as today, social isolation and exclusion are practiced to control the spread of plagues, which protects the community but may cause the affected person to despair. The texts' elitist nature also indicates how socioeconomic factors have always shaped people's experiences of and possibilities to tackle illness.

Meanwhile, two biblical narratives, the tale of Sarai and Abram in Egypt and the mythical exodus, put forward a different perspective on plagues, as their take on them is even celebratory. In these tales, plagues sent by YHWH, the divine puppet master, create horror and hence an escape from a tricky situation. The fictive tales reveal how a specific misfortune can harm some and benefit others, just as the impact of COVID-19 varied drastically, ranging from exposure to health risks (e.g., societally critical jobs) to unexpected travel opportunities (e.g., distance work from the comfort of a summer house). Despite the great temporal and cultural distance, the Hebrew Bible invites us to acknowledge and explore these timeless inequalities in ways how plagues treat people.

Notes

1 This research was enabled by the European Research Council grant 948264 (ANINAN). Thanks are due to Sravana Borkataky-Varma, Christian Eberhart, Marianne Bjelland Kartzow, and Rosanne Liebermann for their helpful comments on earlier versions of this article and to the participants of the Aarhus-McMaster workshop on "Ancient Perspectives on Health and Illness" who discussed the question of social isolation with me.
2 All the English translations of the Hebrew Bible are from *JPS Hebrew-English Tanakh*, with occasional modifications.
3 See Pietrabissa and Simpson, "Isolation;" Seabra et al., *Pandemics*.
4 I agree with the Hebrew word נגע (*nega'*), as well as the related terms, being translated as "plague" broadly understood.
5 E.g., Deut 7:15–20; 2 Sam 24:10–17; 2 Chr 21:12–15. See also Hab 3:5 on YHWH's lethal power.
6 E.g., Exod 15:26; Deut 28:58–63; Zech 14:12–19. On plagues as anticipated future horrors, see also Lev 26:25; Jer 24:10; 29:17; Ezek 38:22; Zech 14:12–18; cf. 2 Chr 6:28; 7:13.
7 See, e.g., Num 8:19; 2 Sam 24:21–25; 1 Kgs 8:37–38; Ps 91:5–6.
8 Following Kleinman (*Patients*, 72), I use the terms "illness" and "disease" as follows: "*Disease* refers to a malfunctioning of biological and/or psychological processes, while the term *illness* refers to the psychosocial experience and meaning of perceived disease." This distinction discourages one from making diagnoses with modern Western biases; Avalos, *Illness*, 27.
9 See Broida, "Medicine," n.p.
10 The lack of seasonal rains was the most typical cause of famines in Canaan. Some texts mention famines owing to natural catastrophes (Deut 28:38–40, 42; Joel 1–2) or political sieges (2 Kgs 6:25; 25:3). In Genesis, the motif signals that living in the promised land is not easy (12:10; 26:1; 42:1–3; 43:1–2); Sarna, *Genesis*, 93.
11 Cf. Gen 20:1–18; 26:1–18 on the motif of presenting one's wife as one's sister.
12 Note the wordplay: another meaning of the root נגע (*n-g-'*), "to plague" or "to afflict," is "to come into physical contact with" or "to harass sexually." See Sarna, *Genesis*, 97.
13 On the sex work motif, see Strine, "Matriarchs," 54–58.
14 See Strine, "Matriarchs," 53–66; idem, "Jacob," 485–498; idem, "Joseph," 55–69.
15 Sarna, *Genesis*, 93.
16 The final form of the plague narrative combines priestly and non-priestly material; Zevit, "Plague," 193–211.
17 Alternatively, the ten calamities could be interpreted as consisting of five pairs of terrors that pertain to the Nile River (1–2), are insects (3–4), comprise diseases (5–6), represent calamities devouring crops (7–8), and pertain to darkness (9–10);

Rendsburg, "Exodus," 114. In any event, the seemingly mild plague of darkness has puzzled scholars. Its effects may include blindness and lameness, which would explain why it was regarded as a devastating force; Moss and Stackert, "Disability," 362–372.

18 On the coercive purpose, see, e.g., Exod 3:20; 6:1; 7:2, 16, 26; 8:16; 9:1, 13; 10:3, 7. On YHWH as the defeater of the Egyptian deities, see Exod 9:14; 12:12; 15:11; 18:11; Num 33:4.

19 See Josh 24:5; 1 Sam 4:8; Amos 4:10; Pss 78:40–51; 105:23–38.

20 Sarna, *Exodus*, 45. On boils, see also Lev 13:18–23.

21 All these stories appear in Numeri. In Num 11:31–34, a plague is sent after a wind blows tons of quails to the camp of the Hebrews who gather more than they can eat. Soon after, the spies sent to explore Canaan die owing to a plague after they had urged people to rebel against Moses (14:36–38). The rebellion of Korah, Datan, and Abiram provokes yet another divine punishment: the earth swallows them (16:31–22), whilst a plague hits the Hebrews (17:12–15). Finally, a plague hits the Hebrews worshipping Baal-Peor (25:8, 18; cf. Ps 106:28–30).

22 Sir 38:1–8, on the contrary, praises physicians as YHWH's collaborators. Medical themes are generally more prominent in early Jewish writings. Jub 10:10–14 even refers to Noah's book of medical knowledge, the only medical work mentioned in Jewish texts. See Hezser, "Physician," 173–197; Askin, *Scribal Culture*, 186–231.

23 In addition, various references point to the existence of physicians (Gen 50:2; Jer 8:22; Job 13:4; 2 Chr 16:12–13). On prayer and healing, see also Gen 20:17; Pss 6:3; 30:3; 41:5; 103:3; 107:20; 147:3.

24 Moss and Schipper, "Introduction," 3.

25 Avalos, *Illness*, 366.

26 Levine, *Leviticus*, xiv, 75.

27 See esp. 2 Chr 23:19 and Avalos, *Illness*, 302, 321–326.

28 Levine, *Leviticus*, xiv.

29 Levine, *Leviticus*, 75. Lev 13:47–59 and 14:33–53 specify that procedures should take place if similar symptoms appear in cloth, leather, or building stones, whereas Lev 14:54–57 provides a postscript to the laws in chs. 13–14; ibid., xiv, 84.

30 See also Lev 13:9, 20, 25, 27, 47, 59; Deut 24:8.

31 The association goes back to the Septuagint, which translates *tsara'at* with λέπρα (*lepra*). Yet the latter means "scaly condition," while ελεφαντίασις (*elephantiasis*) is used of "leprosy" in ancient Greek; Milgrom, *Leviticus*, 775.

32 See Milgrom, *Leviticus*, 775; Avalos, *Illness*, 315.

33 Olyan, *Disability*, 47, 54, 60. The criteria for determining a "defect" remain obscure, but at least the majority of them were regarded as permanent or long lasting; ibid., 28–29. Meanwhile, *tsara'at* is often temporary.

34 On the "sacred-medical" use of the term in Lev 13–14 and Deut 24:8, see Seybold, *Kranken*, 25.

35 Hereafter, the text continues with sections on chronic ailments (13:9–17), *tsara'at* as a secondary development (13:18–46), and *tsara'at* in fabrics and leather (13:47–59); Levine, *Leviticus*, 78–84.

36 It is not apparent why such a condition is regarded as a cause of extreme impurity (cf. Lev 13:45–46). A likely answer is that *tsara'at* causes a state involving the decay of flesh, which creates an association with death (cf. Num 12:10–12), and corpses were regarded as impure (cf. Num 19:11–22); Avalos, *Illness*, 306.

37 The text does not specify whether the isolation is against the person's will, but the use of the verb סגר (*s-g-r*) suggests that her or his movement is restricted (cf. Ezek 3:24).

38 On this view, see, e.g., Marx, "*Lévitique*," 415–433; Smith-Christopher, *Landless*, 144.

39 On the smooth skin as a priestly ideal, see Raphael, *Corpora*, 37; van der Zwan, "Skin," 8.
40 Van der Zwan, "Skin," 3, 9. The heightened focus on purity was perhaps a mechanism of survival for a minority seeking to maintain its distinctive identity under turbulent sociopolitical circumstances; Smith-Christopher, *Landless*, 149. On the postexilic date of Leviticus' final form, see Gerstenberger, *Leviticus*, 12.
41 Raphael, *Corpora*, 38.
42 Walls, "Disability," 25–26.
43 Sweeney, *I & II Kings*, 312.
44 In 2 Kgs 15:5, YHWH is said to hit the king with a plague (נגע, *nega'*), and the ruler is then characterized as suffering from a skin ailment (מצרע, *metsora'*). The account in 2 Chron 26:19–21 refers to how the king got a skin ailment (צרעת, *tsara'at*), and he is also characterized as מצרע (*metsora'*). On the theme of skin ailment as a penalty for transgression, see Olyan, *Disability*, 55–56; Cranz, *Illness*, 115, 163–170.
45 The exact meaning of a "separate house" (בבית החפשית, *bet hakhafshit*) is unclear. It was translated as "in the house of isolation" (ἐν οἴκῳ αφφουσωθ, *en oikō aphphousōth*) in the Septuagint. It has been argued that the term stands for lifelong quarantine, means the physical quarters in which the king lived, or refers to how the king was set free from his royal duties; Cranz, *Illness*, 165n4. The idea of isolated living is plausible in any event.
46 Olyan, "Self," 40–41.
47 Similarly, Avalos, *Illness*, 257.
48 See Seybold, *Kranken*, 98–164. Regarding illness and recovery, see Isa 38:9–20 (cf. 2 Kgs 20); Ps 102:3–4.
49 See also Pss 6, 32, 51, 102, 130, and 143. The first unequivocal grouping of the penitential psalms dates back to Cassiodorus' Commentary on the Psalms from the sixth century CE; Astell, "Psalms," 37–75.
50 On the mixture of distress in Ps 38, see Avalos, *Illness*, 257; Raphael, *Corpora*, 110–114.
51 Cf. Thucydides, *History* 2.51, who comments on how people were afraid of visiting each other during the plague (νόσος, *nosos*) that ravaged Athens in 430/429 BCE, though he also notes how some made it "a point of honour to visit their friends without sparing themselves" (trans. C. F. Smith, Loeb Classical Library 108: 351).
52 While this article has focused on the Hebrew Bible, note that the rabbinic literature of late antiquity discusses the topic at times. Bava Kama 60b offers the advice to stay at home during a plague, while visiting the sick is appreciated according to Nedarim 40a.

Works Cited

Askin, Lindsey A., *Scribal Culture in Ben Sira* (JSJSup 184), Leiden: Brill, 2018.

Astell, Ann W., "Cassiodorus's Commentary on the Psalms as an Ars Rhetorica," *Rhetorica* 17 (1999): 37–75.

Avalos, Hector, *Illness and Health Care in the Ancient Near East: The Role of the Temple in Greece, Mesopotamia, and Israel* (HSM 54), Atlanta: Scholars Press, 1995.

Broida, Marian, "Medicine and the Hebrew Bible," n.p., online: https://www.bibleodyssey.org/en/people/related-articles/medicine-and-the-hebrew-bible (cited 19 January 2022).

Cranz, Isabel, *Royal Illness and Kingship Ideology in the Hebrew Bible* (SOTSMS), Cambridge: Cambridge University Press, 2021.

Gerstenberger, Erhard S., *Das dritte Buch Mose: Leviticus* (ATD 6), Göttingen: Vandenhoeck & Ruprecht, 1993.

Hezser, Catherine, "Representations of the Physician in Jewish Literature from Hellenistic and Roman Times," in *Popular Medicine in Graeco-Roman Antiquity: Explorations*, edited by William V. Harris (Columbia Studies in the Classical Tradition 42), Leiden: Brill, 2016, 173–197.

JPS Hebrew-English Tanakh, Philadelphia: JPS, 2003.

Kleinman, Arthur, *Patients and Healers in the Context of Culture: An Exploration of the Borderland between Anthropology, Medicine, and Psychiatry* (Comparative Studies of Health Systems and Medical Care 3), Berkeley: University of California Press, 1980.

Levine, Baruch A., *Leviticus* (The JPS Torah Commentary), Philadelphia: JPS, 1989.

Marx, Alfred, "Les recherches sur le *Lévitique* et leur impact théologique," *Bib* 88 (2007): 415–433.

Milgrom, Jacob, *Leviticus 1–16: A New Translation with Introduction and Commentary* (AB 3), New York: Doubleday, 1991.

Moss, Candida R. and Jeremy Schipper, "Introduction," in *Disability Studies and Biblical Literature*, edited by Candida R. Moss and Jeremy Schipper, New York: Palgrave Macmillan, 2011, 1–11.

Moss, Candida R. and Jeffrey Stackert, "The Devastation of Darkness: Disability in Exodus 10:21–23, 27, and Intensification in the Plagues," *JR* 92 (2012): 362–372.

Olyan, Saul M., *Disability in the Hebrew Bible: Interpreting Mental and Physical Differences*, New York: Cambridge University Press, 2008.

Olyan, Saul M., "The Search for the Elusive Self in Texts of the Hebrew Bible," in *Religion and the Self in Antiquity*, edited by David Brakke et al., Bloomington: Indiana University Press, 2005, 40–50.

Pietrabissa, Giada and Susan G. Simpson, "Psychological Consequences of Social Isolation during COVID-19 Outbreak," *Front Psychol* 11 (2020): 1–4.

Raphael, Rebecca, *Biblical Corpora: Representations of Disability in Hebrew Biblical Literature* (LHBOTS 445), London: T&T Clark, 2008.

Rendsburg, Gary A., "The Literary Unity of the Exodus Narrative," in *"Did I Not Bring Israel Out of Egypt?" Biblical, Archaeological, and Egyptological Perspectives on the Exodus Narratives*, edited by James K. Hoffmeier et al. (BBRSup 13), Winona Lake: Eisenbrauns, 2016, 113–132.

Sarna, Nahum M., *Exodus* (The JPS Torah Commentary), Philadelphia: JPS, 1991.

Sarna, Nahum M., *Genesis* (The JPS Torah Commentary), Philadelphia: JPS, 1989.

Seabra, Cláudia, Odete Paiva, Carla Silva and José Luís Abrantes, *Pandemics and Travel*, Bingley: Emerald, 2021.

Seybold, Klaus, *Das Gebet des Kranken im Alten Testament: Untersuchungen zur Bestimmung und Zuordnung der Krankheits- und Heilungspsalme* (BWANT 19), Stuttgart: Kohlhammer, 1973.

Smith-Christopher, Daniel L., *The Religion of the Landless: The Social Context of the Babylonian Exile*, Eugene: Wipf & Stock, 2015.

Strine, Casey A., "Sister Save Us: The Matriarchs as Breadwinners and Their Threat to Patriarchy in the Ancestral Narrative," in *Women and Exilic Identity in the Hebrew Bible*, edited by Katherine E. Southwood and Martien A. Halvorson-Taylor (LHBOTS 631), London: Bloomsbury T&T Clark, 2017, 53–66.

Strine, Casey A., "The Famine in the Land Was Severe: Environmentally Induced Involuntary Migration and the Joseph Narrative," *HS* 60 (2019): 55–69.
Strine, Casey A., "The Study of Involuntary Migration as a Hermeneutical Guide for Reading the Jacob Narrative," *BibInt* 26 (2018): 485–498.
Sweeney, Marvin A., *I & II Kings: A Commentary* (OTL), Louisville: Westminster John Knox Press, 2007.
Walls, Neal H., "The Origins of the Disabled Body: Disability in Mesopotamia," in *This Abled Body: Rethinking Disabilities in Biblical Studies*, edited by Hector Avalos et al. (SemeiaSt 55), Atlanta: SBL, 2007, 13–30.
Zevit, Ziony, "The Priestly Redaction and Interpretation of the Plague Narrative in Exodus," *JQR* 66 (1976): 193–211.
Zwan, Pieter van der, "Some Psychoanalytical Meanings of the Skin in Leviticus 13–14," *Verbum et Ecclesia* 37 (2016): 1–10.

10 The Leper as Transcestor

Queens in Exile

Audrey Gale Hall

> וידבר יהוה אל־משה לאמר:
>
> יהוה [YHVH] spoke to Moses [Moshe], saying:
>
> צו את־בני ישראל וישלחו מן־המחנה כל־צרוע וכל־זב וכל טמא לנפש:
>
> Instruct the Israelites to remove from camp anyone with an eruption (*tsarua'*, leprous) or a discharge (*zav*, flow) and anyone defiled by a corpse.
>
> מזכר עד־נקבה תשלחו אל־מחוץ למחנה תשלחום ולא יטמאו את־מחניהם אשר אני שכן בתוכם:
>
> Remove male and female alike; put them outside the camp so that they do not defile the camp of those in whose midst I dwell.
>
> ויעשו־כן בני ישראל וישלחו אותם אל־מחוץ למחנה כאשר דבר יהוה אל־משה כן עשו בני ישראל:
>
> The Israelites did so, putting them outside the camp; as יהוה had spoken to Moses, so the Israelites did.[1]

In the first four verses of chapter 5 in *B^e^midbar* (or the Book of Numbers in English Bible editions), Moshe cleans out the riffraff, certain Israelite bodies which have begun to displease the deity YHVH (יהוה). As the people of Israel wander through the Sinai into Canaan, some have committed such pesky acts as giving birth and menstruating, ejaculating and dripping with other discharges, and developing marks on their skin known as *nega'im tsara'at* (strikings of leprosy). The deity instructs Moshe, one of three siblings he has appointed to lead the twelve tribes, to expel them outside the camp. And just like that, out goes a host of postpartum birthing parents, people with STDs (sexually transmitted disease), everyone on their period, and those who've recently ejaculated. Along with them, oddly enough, are the lepers. While after a time the majority of defiled bodies can be reintegrated into the fold of Hebrew religion, this latter group remains outside the camp with no expiry date.

In this chapter, I take the position that biblical narratives of expulsion and community cause the religious and sexual undertones of *tsara'at* (leprosy) to resonate deeply with contemporary practices of transcestor veneration. In many faith institutions which do not explicitly value trans lives, trans

DOI: 10.4324/b22930-13

experiences in faith institutions include safety risks from passive social exclusion to physical violence, incarceration, and forced houselessness. Increasingly, transgender people have responded to crises of spiritual alienation by building devotional practices around transgender ancestors or transcestors: our communities' elders, martyrs, prophet/esses, saints, and visionaries.

Trans theologians from Jewish and Christian traditions have identified transcestors in specific characters, archetypal figures, and broad historical categories of people from our varying texts and traditions. We are still coming to terms, quite literally, with how the less-than-a-century-year-old U.S. transgender movements carry forth legacies of butches, drag queens, and other gender deviants. I'm writing this chapter to add lepers to their ranks.

1 Outside the Camp

B^e^midbar's sparse, four-verse account of the expulsion of defiled bodies ends with an affirmation that "the Israelites" did as Moses instructed regarding "them," the riffraff I mentioned above. The narrative characteristically depicts the "people of Israel" as a unified actor, not individuals. They respond as one to divine messages issued through a prophet—even removing their own friends and relatives from the midst of the people.

The text does not indicate whether or not anyone flinched at the task of exiling their friends and kinfolk. In fact, it avoids the question altogether. The reader of *B^e^midbar* is never told what happened to that first round of people removed from the camp. Immediately after verse 4, the priestly voice abruptly transitions to a seemingly unrelated conversation about reparation offerings in cases of interpersonal harm between Israelites: "And YHVH spoke to Moshe, saying..." (5:5). The text never again mentions any horde dripping with fluid, nor does its narrative voice follow the exiles to the outer edges of their nation. They disappear through cracks in the story, in the space between verses 4 and 5.

This piece of *B^e^midbar* is attributed to the Priestly Source, a theologically and stylistically unique body of scripture including *Vayikra* (or the book of Leviticus), which contains most of the legal statutes in the Torah. In *Vayikra*, the deviance of certain human and animal forms is codified with the word *tumah* (האמוט), or "defilement."

Besides lepers, other defiled people are not to be kept out in perpetuity but instead must fulfill timebound ritual obligations in order to enter *taharah* (טהרה), a status of ritual eligibility often translated as "cleanness" or "purity." For example, *Vayikra* chapter 12 specifies that whereas menstruation is a *tame'* (defiled) state, postpartum *tumah* lasts one or two weeks, depending on whether a child is male or female.

After this period of time follows one or two months wherein the birthing parent remains "in the blood of her purifying" and cannot enter the sanctuary. A priest may offer the appropriate animal sacrifices on the parent's behalf, whereupon "she shall be clean" (Lev 12:1–8). In this sense, *tumah* not only describes a spiritual state of being but also pronounces a taboo, prescribes actions and counter-actions, and inscribes otherness.

At the time of *B^emidbar* 5, there is no precedent recorded in scripture regarding these leaky, pustular bodies who birth and menstruate and orgasm, flake and ooze and peel. The purity laws of *Vayikra* 11–15 clearly mandate that anyone who develops *tsara'at* (leprosy) leave the camp promptly upon diagnosis (13:46). Because lepers are present to be expelled in *B^emidbar* 5:1, the passage can chronologically be placed before that.

So menstruating people, like *metsora'im*, are *tame'* during the time of their flow. However, of the two groups, only lepers are kept outside the camp without end date. Besides leprosy, one other permanent ban exists in scripture with regards to bodily *tumah*—*Vayikra* specifies that participating in period sex should result in someone being "cut off from among their people" (Lev 20:18). Thus, sexual stigma is reinforced against bodies who bleed, just as later rabbinic instructions would restrict the sexuality of *metsora'im*. At the time of *B^emidbar* 5, however, there are no such recorded legal statutes in place.

Before the laws come into effect, much of the community is expelled while others, referred to collectively as the "people of Israel," actively participate in their removal at Moshe's instruction. Does anyone object or resist? Are the expelled not also people of Israel? Their exile does not apparently end; the people are never said to return, and their side of the story is not represented in the form of challenges, protestations, or a refusal to comply. A reader of *B^emidbar* may assume that YHVH gave an immediate follow-up order allowing some or all of the folks to return. Or maybe Aharon, Miriam, or Moshe intervened with reports of a new revelation in favor of the exiles, resolving the tension left palpably present in the text and allowing them to re-enter the community.

But there is just as much evidence to support an assumption that at least for some amount of time, nobody did anything and YHVH became silent. The wind died down, people remembered their daily tasks, and life went on. In this case, the defiled people are left for days, months, or years at the margins of the camp, severed from a familiar rhythm of festivities, meals, prayers, and rituals. They may have smelled their cousins' offerings of incense and meat, heard familiar melodies, and watched smoke waft toward heaven. However, they would not be permitted to worship at the tent of meeting, would not access the altar, and would not be acceptable in the divine presence.

At some point after this story, YHVH delivers the purity laws, which set allotted times after which *some* categories of defiled people would have the ability to return. I can imagine a traumatized collection of people, many still aching from birth and menses, urinary tract infections, and skin lesions, aching for a chance to bathe again, trickling back into the camp, unable to trust their god, prophet, or people to care for them. They would slowly reintegrate, to an extent, into their community of origin, grasping for reasons to believe that YHVH would not reject them again.

And, unfortunately for those bearing the mark of leprosy, they are prescribed a unique ritual role as the only Israelites who can never be touched, the physical embodiment of the boundary between the community of YHVH and the outer world. The leper exemplifies and makes clear that some bodies are eligible while others are not. In this text, they are referred to with an adjective— "the leprous" (*hatsarua'*)—but more often than not, *Vayikra* refers to their body only in terms of a *tame'* blemish known as the *nega' tsara'at.*[2] Later on, rabbinic Hebrew develops the term *metsora* for someone who has leprosy, which more easily translates as "leper."

Thus, *B^{e}midbar* 5 features an origin story and narrative precedent for the particular system of bodily surveillance laid out in the purity laws of *Vayikra.* Transgender theologian Joy Ladin identifies the familiar experience of "gender surveillance—the ongoing scrutiny of bodies, clothing, voices, and gestures to determine if we are male or female."[3] She compares the removal of lepers and other stigmatized people to the transphobic trend of "bathroom bills," which encourage scrutiny of bodies who appear gender-non-compliant in the place they wish to defecate. Ladin suggests that although the Torah does not acknowledge people outside the male-female gender binary, *Vayikra's* legislation concerning lepers should compel modern Jewish communities to address the personal and systemic transphobia that leads "so many of us [trans people] to be removed, or to remove ourselves, from the camp."[4]

As evidenced by the inclusion of lepers among people in the midst of sexual functions, sexuality, gender, and *tsara'at* ought not be considered mutually exclusive aspects of human life from a biblical perspective. Here, I must invoke queer philosopher Michel Foucault's theory of the "discourse": a social system that creates meaning, which in turn shapes the physical world and its social systems. In his massive *History of Sexuality*, Foucault traces the emergence of "sexuality" as a concept produced by discourses in Victorian-era sexology, around the time that new terms such as "homosexual" emerged to define human sexual beings by their human sexual doings. Cultural discourses reinforce the material world through acts of language, "practices that systematically form the objects of which they speak."[5]

A discourse on lepers creates lepers. For example, take *Vayikra* 13, which mostly consists of a verbal flowchart for religious professionals called *kohanim* (often called priests) to diagnose *tsara'at.* The text instructs the *kohen* to examine a potential leper and then make an official proclamation of whether they are *tame'* or *tahor* (ritually eligible). This speech act transitions *metsora'im* from one ritual state to another, which results in banishment from the community. Think about all that can follow when a person comes out, or *is outed*, as transgender. Suddenly their transness, like *tsara'at*, becomes a publicly known quality, out of their control, which brings social consequences—positive, negative, and neutral. In this sense, both gender and leprous defilement get tied up with cultural systems of meaning and are not biological constants.

I say "not biological constants" because I want to point out that *tsara'at* is not a clear medical concept. It is a religious, semi-magical phenomenon that grows on people's skin, on houses, on fabric. The diagnosis also includes symptoms from a number of different diseases, and does not match up with anything known to modern science. It does not seem like *tsara'at* has an epidemiological unity to it in any way. So, by creating laws on the basis of this unstable category, *Vayikra* produces a new discourse where *tsara'at* is a real thing that the authorities can then identify and remove.

The measures prescribed in *Vayikra* provide for the removal of leprous bodies and objects from the midst of the people, outside of the community. And yet the text never connects theological dots between the three manifestations of *tsara'at* on humans, fabric items, and buildings. Their conceptual relationship remains unspecified. The only uniting factor is the priest's role: determining whether the substance is or is not *tsara'at*, verbally declaring it to be defiling (*tame'*) or not (*tahor*), then seeing to the removal of any defiling person or item from the community.

2 Trauma Response: Exile or Exit?

In light of the broad diversity of political circumstances and religious traditions which trans people inherit, transform, and experience, I want to be clear about who I am interpreting for. That is, for myself, a transsexual raised by WASPs, or White Anglo-Saxon Protestants, in suburban North Texas during the 2000s and 2010s.[6] Incidentally (and by design), academic literature on the subject of trans spirituality tends to prioritize white and Christian and American concerns and research participants. So although I maintain that leprous transcestors can present a valuable theological resource for Jews, Christians of color, Catholics, and all others who draw on the Bible for inspiration, in this article I will remain primarily in my own lane.

Lately, entire denominations of American Christianity have boiled and fractured over whether to tolerate the bodies of LGBTQI2+ people in their pews or pulpits, whether to allow us to meaningfully take part in the global communion of believers, and whether to designate queer families as either sacramental or blasphemous.[7] Queer theologian Marcella Althaus-Reid calls this the hegemony of western imperial and patriarchal theology: that normative "sexual Christology" has exclusively settled on the nuclear family unit as the only form of economic, sexual, and social organization permitted by the divine.[8] In this sense, heteronormative Christianity, as well as individual actors within spiritual communities, contribute directly to the premature deaths of LGBTQI2+ people.

Among cis-heterosexual Americans for whom dominant religious institutions are designed, engagement with organized religion is "typically protective against suicide." However, the opposite is true of LGB folks, for whom religious experiences generally increase the likelihood of suicidal ideation and attempts.[9] For transgender people, especially trans women, higher degrees of participation in religious institutions have been found to correlate with higher levels of mental health problems as well as riskier sexual activity.[10]

One American study found that trans and gender non-conforming identities could be used to predict religious and spiritual struggles empirically linked to depression, anxiety, lower self-esteem, and lower trait resilience. In the study, which disproportionately sampled white TGNC participants from Christian households, 41% of TGNC respondents reported attempting suicide, over 30 times the figure for the general American population (1.2%).[11] The researchers found that more than half of transgender people who had been religiously affiliated at one time or another reported experiencing rejection in religious communities. This pattern coincides with a "massive exit" of TGNC people from organized religious communities, leaving fewer than 20% of transgender respondents engaged in organized religion at the time of the study.[12] As Ladin indicates, the "massive exit" must be understood in terms of both voluntary departures and communal exclusion.

Trans folks who remain in religious communities may experience their religious life narrative as bittersweet, not entirely traumatic, and containing valuable elements we can reclaim and continue to utilize. For example, social science researchers point out that even while simultaneously coping with "some family members' attempts to use religion to shame them," transgender participants commonly reported that "their personal religious and spiritual practices were integral to their resilience."[13]

Walker and Longmire-Avital found that especially among Black LGB individuals "at the margins of racial and sexual discrimination ... use of religion as a coping tool is a common practice."[14] On a surface level, these findings appear contradictory to other research presenting religious involvement as a mitigating factor in TGNC emotional health. But rather than clashing, this variety of patterns reflects a diversity in religious experience across American trans populations, mediated by factors including denomination, gender identity, and racialized experiences.

Churches and Christian families frequently exacerbate the issue by rejecting their trans members. The impacts are disproportionately born by those of us who cannot provide our own housing: poor and disabled trans people, our elders, our youth. The majority of cis-heterosexual Americans of faith accept this dynamic, whether enthusiastically or by tacit consent. Indeed, transprejudice was found in an analysis of three dozen studies to correlate with measures of religiosity, i.e., religious attendance, religious self-identification, and fundamentalism.[15] These findings are also based on research overrepresenting white Christians, the authors acknowledge. So perhaps it is more specifically accurate to conclude that higher religiosity among white cisgender Christian Americans correlates with hostility toward trans folks, whether or not they have ever knowingly interacted with one of us.

The multiple spiritual impacts of gender marginalization on trans folks are collectively known as religious abuse, defined as the experience of psychological distress following "condemnation, rejection, or guilt." This cultural matrix of harm "damages LGBT individuals' spirituality, creating incongruence and cognitive dissonance related to religious and sexual identities."[16] And like many cultural processes, anti-trans religious abuse relies on commonly held language and expectations around gender in order to function.

3 Lineages of Deviance

I first heard the word "transcestor," a portmanteau of "transgender" and "ancestor," during the opening ceremony of the ninth Southern Movement Assembly (SMA 9), held on Zoom in September 2020. The SMA called on our forebears, trans as well as cis, as we convened folks representing frontlines, organizations, and people's movement assemblies from across the U.S. South. My comrade Nathalie Nia Faulk led a hundred or so Southern activists through a centering ritual in which she called on social movement "ancestors and transcestors," named and unnamed, whose love and struggle prepared the way for our own. In one word, "transcestors," Nathalie Nia passed on a powerful tool I had yet to encounter.

As a mode of spiritual engagement, transcestor veneration responds to the unique spiritual and survival needs of trans communities abandoned to AIDS, houselessness, incarceration, police violence, sexual violence, and death from suicide. Trans people of faith, and those of us with no faith, have to deal with the role played by violent theologies in our various public health crises. Of course, before SMA 9, I knew the names of some of the gender non-conforming people who paved the way for myself and my queer siblings, but I had yet to understand any of their stories as components of a lineage with which I could be in relationship.

The idea of transcestry was introduced to trans biblical interpreter Lewis Reay by "a young transman," uncredited, who I presume learned it in a community setting much as myself.[17] In his 2009 essay "Towards a Transgender Theology: Que(e)rying the Eunuchs," Reay argues that intersex and transgender interpreters can understand the eunuch in Acts 8 as a spiritual transcestor, along with 23 other eunuch figures in biblical literature, including the bonus addition of Jesus himself, whom Reay dubs a "gender queer, virgin born, intersex, transman."[18] Such deliciously subversive language could confuse even a devout transgender Christian. It may seem provocative or theologically ungrounded. Yet in fact, Reay was expounding from an established body of queer theological scholarship regarding eunuchs and intersexuality, the gender and sexual deviance of Jesus, and a transgender God.[19] Since 2009, a number of published anthologies and online compilations have highlighted written contributions to the field of transcestor veneration, utilizing the term at times and, at others (especially before 2009), simply living it out.[20]

At the same time as—and centuries prior to—Reay's work on the eunuch from his Christian perspective, Jewish authors in particular have addressed the presence of trans and intersex bodies among the people of Israel. As early as the 2nd century CE, rabbinic authors acknowledged several configurations of sex and gender in addition to the *man* and the *woman*: "not only … the *androginos* (a [person] with both male and female sexual organs) but also of the *tumtum* (with hidden or undeveloped genitals), the *aylonit* (a masculine or infertile woman), and the *saris* (a feminine or infertile man)."[21]

And yet from a conservative sexual-theological perspective, gender non-conforming people's existence may appear to violate an otherwise orderly and categorizable creation. Jewish feminist theologian Judith Plaskow includes transgender/intersex embodiment among those anomalies which "endanger the foundations of the earth" from certain vantage points nestled within patriarchy.[22] The conflation of feminized and sexualized body conditions with leprosy establishes clear links to theologies that condemn sexual pleasure and gender autonomy.

The recovery of transcestors in one's own sacred texts and traditions is, as Rabbi Elliot Kukla writes, a spiritual sort of homecoming. Kukla argues that given the literal and spiritual homelessness of so many trans communities, the holiness of ancient exceptions to the gender/sex binary "indicates an opening toward infinite locations for belonging that are still authentically connected to our histories and communities."[23]

Although Reay may have been first to set "transcestor" to print, I identify Leslie Feinberg's book *Transgender Warriors: Making History from Joan of Arc to Dennis Rodman* as the earliest written and published work of transcestor veneration. Although Feinberg did not use that terminology nor Reay's explicitly Christian framing. Rather, hir book challenged members of nascent American transgender movements to understand their interconnectedness with others across space and time. Feinberg recorded stories by Two-Spirit people and body-builder cis women, hijras, and "bearded ladies," all of whose lives attest to the continuity and viability of life outside the strictest western binary of manhood and womanhood. Feinberg's history was aimed at "not *defining* but *defending*" emergent trans communities writ large at a tender moment in their coalescence. Zie declared hir intent "to fashion history, politics, and theory into a steely weapon with which to defend a very oppressed segment of the population."[24] In this sense, *Transgender Warriors* is not merely a book but also an act of political resistance, echoing the bricks thrown at Stonewall. I count Feinberg, who passed away in 2014, a transcestor in hir own right.

The narrative frame of transcestry provides avenues through which trans people can deepen our ongoing work of joy, resistance, and survival by celebrating the resilience of our elders and dreaming a world into being in which our descendants can thrive. Writing to a medieval studies audience on the topic of "premodern trans histories," M. W. Bychowski and Dorothy Kim explain the value of reading historical texts for glimpses of transgressive gender and sexual embodiment:

> … by saying that trans people have an acknowledged past, trans people can better imagine a future. In this way, our work on the past is to tell

> the story of trans lives for the political, intersectional, and community aims of building a future for trans lives now. ... It is worth pausing to consider all the things we might have been shown and all the ways we might have learned to see if only our histories, our societies, and our political choices better supported those we have lost.[25]

As Bychowski and Kim reach far back to reveal transgressive gender in stories from medieval Europe, I have already demonstrated one instance in which Jewish and Christian trans people may also stretch ourselves toward biblical lineages of leprosy to find kinship and spiritual ancestry. The first generation of lepers, those who found themselves expelled in *Beᵉmidbar* 5, may resonate with trans people's yearning to know our deeper roots. At least in the Torah, they were the first of their kind. Admittedly, in one earlier story, Moshe himself received *tsara'at* on his hand, as a momentary demonstration of YHVH's power, which was hastily undone (*Shemot* 4:6–7). And yet no earlier biblical figures are characterized as *hatsarua'* ("the leprous," biblical Hebrew) or *metsora* ("leper," rabbinic Hebrew). So this cohort of outcasts would have developed their own understandings of what it meant to be a leper, ever on the outside.

Without adequate language, cultural structures, or political movements to draw on for meaning, the emergence of new subjugated identities requires grappling with oppressive ideologies that keep freaks in their place. Trans people of the 21st century frequently point to individuals such as Marsha P. Johnson and Sylvia Rivera as forebears and role models, living in a liminal time when "trans" was only on the tip of the collective queer tongue. These drag queens struggled within the gay liberation movement against the dismissal and exclusion of people who crossed gender lines, houseless people, people of color, and others within the umbrella of Gay Liberation who were nevertheless shoved out into the rain.

Rivera famously referred to herself and others in the organization Street Transvestite Action Revolutionaries (STAR) as "half sisters and half brothers of the revolution," a moniker alluding to the partialness of transitional gender identity as well as the status of street queens as both inside and outside the gay movement, depending on the whims of white, economically secure, respectable, and professional activists. Disowned as a child by her conservative Catholic grandmother (and sole guardian), Rivera describes how her experience as a "Queen in Exile" had been thoroughly characterized by the *novelty* of communal gender deviance in a world where "transgender" was not yet a household phrase:

> I didn't really come out as a drag queen until the late 60s, when drag queens were arrested, what degradation there was ... In Spanish cultures, if you're effeminate, you're automatically a fag; you're a gay boy. I mean, you start off as a young child and you don't have an option - especially back then. You were either a fag or a dyke. There was

> no in-between. You have your journey through society the way it is structured. That's how I fit into it at that time in my life. Those were the words of that era. I was an effeminate gay boy. I was becoming a beautiful drag queen, a beautiful drag-queen child. ... We had cross-dressers, but I didn't even know what cross-dressers were until much later. ... People now want to call me a lesbian because I'm with Julia [Murray, Rivera's partner], and I say, "No. I'm just me. I'm not a lesbian." I'm tired of being labeled. I don't even like the label *transgender*. I'm tired of living with labels. I just want to be who I am. I am Sylvia Rivera. Ray Rivera left home at the age of 10 to become Sylvia. And that's who I am.[26]

In that year, at the age of ten, Rivera found herself taken under the wings of other young drag queens who had been "roaming from house to house" and selling sex to survive. Over the next several decades, along with Marsha P. Johnson and others in STAR, she developed a spiritual and communal orientation toward survival, based on an audacious "refashioning of medieval cults of sainthood."[27] In one interview, she shared a liturgical format:

> We'd all get together to pray to our saints before we'd go out hustling. A majority of the queens were Latin and we believe in an emotional, spiritualistic religion. We have our own saints: Saint Barbara, the patron saint of homosexuality, St. Michael, the Archangel; La Caridad de Cobre, the Madonna of gold; and Saint Martha, the saint of transformation. St. Martha had once transformed herself into a snake, so to her we'd pray: "Please don't let them see through the mask. Let us pass as women and save us from harm." And to the other three we'd kneel before our altar of candles and pray: "St. Barbara, St. Michael, La Caridad de Cobre: We know we are doing wrong, but we got to live and we got to survive, so please help us, bring us money tonight, protect us, and keep evil away."[28]

Although the word "ancestor" does not appear in Rivera or Johnson's oral histories or written work, to my knowledge, these and other practices exemplify the reclamatory trans instinct toward identification with those who work the street corners, who roam the wilderness beyond the tabernacle, whose bodies shift and reshape and ooze. In addition, the reappropriation of figures such as saints and angels and Rivera's ritual engagement with them as sources of protection offers a model of theological revisionism to trans folks who choose to remain in religious institutions and other environments hostile to our bodies and spirits. Half-sisters and half-brothers, too, may theologize.

If saints and angels are on the table for trans interpretation and prayerful engagement, how much more are lepers *off* the table and thus uniquely apropos subjects of veneration for queens in exile—and, I must add, kings and nonbinary royalty of all sorts. The gendered and sexualized stigmatization of leprosy lends a critical religious perspective to the ongoing work of stripping down cisheteropatriarchy to its blasphemous underwear. That is, the leper's position alongside menstruating, birthing, and sexually active bodies invites an interrogation of western religious fixation on bodily purity and Christendom's orthodox ordering of men and women along sheer, artificial lines of difference.

This chapter has ventured only a cursory exploration of one among many leper narratives in Hebrew scripture, anchored within a broad stroke, Christian-centric account of transgender spirituality in the United States. By uniting drag queens outside the Israelite camp with lepers outside Stonewall Inn, I hope this offering weaves a biblical narrative of spiritual solidarity beyond the margins of acceptable religious expression and agitates the leprous or transgender reader to insist on our stories' mutual sacredness.

Notes

1 *Bemidbar* 5:1–4, JPS Tanakh.
2 English translations simplify this confusing language by opting for the word "leper" in keeping with the Greek *lepros* (NKJV), or using variations on person-first language, as in the JPS's "person with a leprous affection" (JPS, NASB, NIV, NRSV).
3 Ladin, "Gender Inside and Outside the Camp."
4 Ibid.
5 Foucault, *The Archaeology of Knowledge*, 54.
6 Trans folks use a wide range of language to describe our bodies, and many have rejected "transsexual" as a baldly medical term originating in psychiatry. These transgender-but-not-transsexual folks are valid and their preferences should be honored. Nevertheless, I use the term for myself alongside others before, contemporary with, and descending from me who choose it. My use of "transsexualism" is a deliberate choice. I'm agender, nonbinary, trans, transfeminine, transgender, transsexual, transvestite — names which shift according to present company and context as well as my stage of life, and state of mind.
7 I use this acronym as an incomplete reference to lesbian, gay, bisexual, transgender, queer or questioning, intersex, and Two Spirit people, plus others of "us" who identify with other letters (and perhaps numbers?) which I do not list for the sake of brevity. I do not yet know of a perfectly agreeable way to name all our communities as one or at once, and am not holding my breath.
8 Althaus-Reid, *Indecent Theology*, 95–96.
9 Lytle et al., "Association of Religiosity," 3. "LGB" indicates lesbian, gay, and bisexual people whom the authors surveyed. Many LGB people are also transgender, nonbinary, intersex, et cetera, but in this context I follow Lytle et al. in referring to minorities of sexual orientation by this shorter acronym.
10 Golub et al., "The role of religiosity," 1136.
11 The authors of the study use "TGNC" to refer to their respondent population of transgender and other gender non-conforming people. As LGB indicates people with marginalized sexual orientations, TGNC indicates people of marginalized gender identities who are not cisgender women or men.
12 Exline, et al., "Religious and Spiritual Struggles," 277–280.
13 Follins, et al., "Resilience in Black LGBT Individuals," 200.
14 Walker and Longmire-Avital, "The Impact of Religious Faith," 1723 and 1727.
15 Campbell, et al., "Religion and Attitudes," 6.
16 Super and Jacobson, quoted in Pruitt, "Spirituality and Wellness," 17.

17 Reay, "Towards a Transgender Theology," 149.
18 Reay, "Towards a Transgender Theology," 154.
19 This scholarly canon has only expanded since then. Reay especially draws on Althaus-Reid, *The Queer God*; Goss, *Jesus Acted Up: A Gay and Lesbian Manifesto*; Mollenkott, *Omnigender*; and Ringrose, *The Perfect Servant: Eunuchs and the Social Construction of Gender in Byzantium.*
20 Examples include dodd's [sic] "Imprecatory Prayer to the Transcestors" in *We Have Never Asked Permission to Sing*; Driskill's "For Marsha (Pay It No Mind!) Johnson"; Edidi's "Temple Hymn to Sex Workers" in *The Black Trans Prayer Book*; and Quito Ziegler's *Transgender Rite of Ancestor Elevation.*
21 Wenig, "Male and Female God Created Them," 15.
22 Plaskow, "Dismantling the Gender Binary within Judaism," 187.
23 Kukla, "A Created Being of Its Own," 7.
24 Feinberg, *Transgender Warriors*, xii–xiii.
25 Bychowski and Kim, "Visions of Medieval Trans Feminism," 10.
26 Rivera, "Queens in Exile," 40–48.
27 Ellison and Hoffman, "The Afterward," 283.
28 Cohen, *An Army of Lovers*, 134.

Works Cited

Althaus-Reid, Marcella, *Indecent Theology: Theological Perversions in Sex, Gender, and Politics,* London: Routledge, 2001.

Althaus-Reid, Marcella, *The Queer God*, London: Routledge, 2003.

Bychowski, M. W., and Dorothy Kim, "Visions of Medieval Trans Feminism: An Introduction," *Medieval Feminist Forum* 55, 1 (2019): 6–41.

Campbell, Marianne, Jordan D. X. Hinton, and Joel R. Andreson, "A Systematic Review of the Relationship between Religion and Attitudes toward Transgender and Gender-Variant People," *International Journal of Transgenderism* 20, 1 (2019): 21–38.

Cohen, Stephan L., *The Gay Liberation Youth Movement in New York: "An Army of Lovers Cannot Fail,"* New York: Routledge, 2008.

dodd, jayy, "Imprecatory Prayer to the Transestors," in *We Have Never Asked Permission to Sing: Poetry Celebrating Trans Resilience*, edited by Kemi Alabi, Oakland: Forward Together, 2019, 15.

Driskill, Qwo-Li, "For Marsha P. (Pay It No Mind!) Johnson," *Lodestar Quarterly* 11 (2004), https://lodestarquarterly.com/work/248/.

Edidi, Lady Dane Figueroa, "A Temple Hymn for Sex Workers," in *The Black Trans Prayer Book*, edited by Dane Figueroa Edidi and J Mase III, Morrisville, NC: Lulu, 2020, 152–159.

Ellison, Joy, and Nicholas Hoffman, "The Afterward: Sylvia Rivera and Marsha P. Johnson in the Medieval Imaginary," *Medieval Feminist Forum* 55, 1 (2019): 267–294.

Exline, Julie J., Amy Przeworski, Emily K. Peterson, Margarid R. Turnamian, Nick Stauner, and Alex Uzdavines, "Religious and Spiritual Struggles Among Transgender and Gender-Nonconforming Adults," *Psychology of Religion and Spirituality* 13, 3 (2021): 276–286.

Feinberg, Leslie, *Transgender Warriors: Making History from Joan of Arc to Dennis Rodman*, Boston: Beacon Press, 1996.

Follins, Lourdes D., Ja'Nina J. Walker, and Michele K. Lewis, "Resilience in Black Lesbian, Gay, Bisexual, and Transgender Individuals: A Critical Review of the Literature," *Journal of Gay & Lesbian Mental Health* 18 (2014): 190–212.

Foucault, Michel, *The Archaeology of Knowledge*, trans. A.M. Sheridan Smith, New York: Pantheon Books, 1972.

Golub, Sarit Al, Ja'Nina J. Walker, Buffie Longmire-Avital, David S. Bimbi, and Jeffrey T. Parsons, "The Role of Religiosity, Social Support, and Stress-Related Growth in Protecting Against HIV Risk among Transgender Women," *Journal of Helath Psychology* 15, 8 (2010): 1135–1144.

Goss, Robert, *Jesus Acted Up: A Gay and Lesbian Manifesto*, San Francisco: Harper Collins, 1994.

Kukla, Elliot, "A Created Being of Its Own: Toward a Jewish Liberation Theology for Men, Women and Everyone Else," *TransTorah*, 2006, http://transtorah.org/PDFs/How_I_Met_the_Tumtum.pdf.

Ladin, Joy, "Gender Inside and Outside the Camp," *Torah Online Commentary*, Jewish Theological Seminary, 2017, https://www.jtsa.edu/torah/gender-inside-and-outside-the-camp/.

Lytle, Megan C., John R. Blosnich, Susan M. De Luca, and Chris Brownson, "Association of Religiosity with Sexual Minority Suicide Ideation and Attempt," *American Journal of Preventive Medicine* 54, 5 (2018): 644–651.

Mollenkott, Virginia Ramey, *Omnigender: A Trans-Religious Approach*, Cleveland: Pilgrim Press, 2001.

Plaskow, Judith, "Dismantling the Gender Binary within Judaism," in *Balancing on the Mechitza: Transgender in Jewish Community*, edited by Noach Dzmura, Berkeley: North Atlantic Books, 2010, 187–210.

Pruitt, Black, "Spirituality & Wellness in the Black LGBTQIA+ Experience: A Literature Review," Expressive Arts Therapy MA thesis, Lesley University, *Expressive Therapies Capstone Theses* 620 (2022): 1–32.

Reay, Lewis, "Towards a Transgender Theology: Que(e)rying the Eunuchs," in *Trans/Formations*, edited by Marcella Althaus-Reid and Lisa Isherwood, Norwich, UK: Hymns Ancient and Modern, 2009, 148–167.

Ringrose, Kathryn M., *The Perfect Servant: Eunuchs and the Social Construction of Gender in Byzantium*, University of Chicago Press, 2007.

Rivera, Sylvia, "Queens in Exile: The Forgotten Ones," in *Street Transvestite Action Revolutionaries: Survival, Revolt, and Queer Antagonist Struggle*, edited by Ehn Nothing, Untorelli Press, 2006, 40–55. Originally published in *GenderQueer: Voices From Beyond the Sexual Binary*, edited by Joan Nestle, Clare Howell, and Riki Wilchins, Alyson Books, 2002, 70–88.

Super, John T., and Lamerial Jacobson, "Religious Abuse: Implications for Counseling Lesbian, Gay, Bisexual, and Transgender Individuals," *Journal of LGBT Issues in Counseling* 5 (2011): 180–196.

Walker, Ja'Nina J., and Buffie Longmire-Avital, "The Impact of Religious Faith and Internalized Homonegativity on Resiliency for Black Lesbian, Gay, and Bisexual Emerging Adults," *Developmental Psychology* 49, 9 (2013): 1723–1731.

Wenig, Margaret Moers, "Spiritual Lessons I Have Learned from Transsexuals," in *Balancing on the Mechitza: Transgender in Jewish Community*, edited by Noach Dzmura, Berkeley: North Atlantic Books, 2010, 60–67.

Ziegler, Quito, aka Forest of the Future, "Prayer to the Ancestors," *Transgender Rite of Ancestor Elevation*, Tumblr, 2013, https://trans-rite.tumblr.com/post/180084347277/prayer-to-the-ancestors-an-invocation-and.

11 Constructing the Sacred Self

21st-Century Paganism, Self-care, and Ascetic Witchcraft

MiloRhys K. Teplin di Padilla

1 Introduction

During the isolation of the lockdown measures enacted throughout the COVID-19 pandemic, practices and ideals stemming from a mantra of "self-care" surged online. Sleeping in, meditation, and purposely not feeling guilty while indulging oneself often are the hallmarks of self-care; however, some aspects of the occult were often tied into this. Tarot card reading, prayer candles, and other forms of mystical self-actualization are prevalent in many spaces that tout spiritual wellness. What causes some people to only adopt occult methodologies briefly while others integrate them as a part of their lives? After all, modern-day occult practices are an amalgamation of religious and philosophical practices, not a fashion item. To answer these questions, we must look a little deeper at not only existing social power structures, but at what religion does. Religion has been referred to as a powerful tool in a variety of contexts, and justifiably so: it is a means to self-empowerment, a framework for contextualizing the unknowable around us, a vibrant social activity, and a means of better connecting with one's heritage. Using these ideas as the lens by which we view the arena of social media forums, we can paint a clearer picture of how paganism as a philosophy has been able to flourish among younger generations.

One must consider ideas of disempowerment in the communities where the trends of self-care and casual occult practices are flourishing. Women, minorities, members of the LGBTQAI+ community, and those from impoverished backgrounds, make up the bulk of those actively engaging in occult pursuits in the study associated with this paper (Teplin 2021). While pagan groups have risen and fallen in popularity over the past century and a half in the global north, the advent of the internet has allowed for the exchange of information to be both easier and more personal. This latest iteration of witchcraft practices has been utilized as a means to better mental health, to foster a sense of self-worth and community, and to deepen one's connection to their genealogical background. This is evident in the noted trend among those who have grown up with internet-based technology and social media having a greater willingness to self-care, open-mindedness, and social

DOI: 10.4324/b22930-14

accountability (Carrier et al. 2015, Howick & Rees 2017, Saunders 2020, Steinert 2021). Feelings of disempowerment and hopelessness during the isolation of trying to survive a global crisis lead naturally to seeking comfort. This may be through enforcing a façade of normalcy among a group of people, to seek guidance from a higher power (whether supernatural or governmental), or to assure oneself that sweeping changes can somehow be made to make all the chaos vanish.

Self-care as a concept is not new, and neither is its connection to the supernatural or even the pseudo-spiritual. Whether found in the Epicureanism of ancient Greece or a popular 2011 episode of the television series "Parks and Rec," mollifying one's own stress through self-indulgence is a pervasive strategy ("Pawnee Rangers" 2011). Many of these models of self-care, mystic or otherwise, hinge on indulgence in a way that feeds into a capitalist model of enjoyment. Colloquially referred to as "retail therapy," the purchase of items to gain a boost of serotonin is a frequent player in discussions of how to best enact self-care (Kang & Johnson 2011, Burke 2018, Lee & Lee 2019). In the accounts from research subjects below, we will see how trends of self-care and goals of self-actualization both drive and reinforce attempts to empower oneself as well as make sense of the random events of the world around them. During this study, the ways in which people approached religious expression often fell into one of two categories: shopping around for a solution model for their needs or strictly seeking to connect with one's heritage. This religious commodification is further reflected in an analysis of how rituals are enacted. In the effort to seek spiritual fulfillment after rejecting more mainstream models, interaction with the supernatural often continues to be materially focused. This is neither a good nor a bad thing; it is merely a means by which we can analyze how the supernatural is contextualized across religions within one overarching cultural system.

What exactly do we mean when we say "commodification" in relation to self-care or religious beliefs? What does this look like in the field? To answer these questions, I would like to analyze a yearly ritual enacted by one study participant in particular. Every fall he would drive a few hours north to some apple orchards that he had deemed particularly beautiful and calming to walk around, pick some apples, and select one to leave as an offering on the altar in his living room. Once the apple had begun to age, he would mash it into a fermented liquor and serve it at a small dinner party where the guests who were aware of this tradition played karaoke. While the study participant spoke of how his yearly ritual was influenced by ideas from pre-Christian Scandinavia—and it clearly was (Rodriguez 2007, Eliferova 2008, Magnell & Iregren 2010)—we can also break this down into more universal terms. The ideas of pilgrimage, material offering, and a religious meal are staples of all religious traditions, especially those that occur during the autumnal/harvest seasons, as this yearly drive does. Even the fact that the study participant takes the time to walk around the orchard in religious contemplation has parallels in Christian monks' walks, Buddhist *kinhin* sessions, and the

Jewish *hakafot*. The acquiring and use of apples in this specific instance is more involved than "buy apples." Providing for one's altar at home is often the extent of pagan worship during the holidays, just as Christians at their church might help purchase costumes for a nativity play. Simple transactions make the process more readily accessible to a wider audience.

In the global north, the self-care movement is a means by which people can focus on their own well-being, in putting their own physical and mental health ahead of the grind of performance, often while nurturing the growth and stability of one's community ahead of material gain. This is radically different from the other predominant viewpoint in the global north: the need to over-achieve and out-perform one's peers and superiors, ensuring the betterment of the individual while attempting to distance oneself from the fate of the collective. The self-care movement as it has been realized within the 21st-century witchcraft community emphasizes this self-actualization as a cornerstone of one's spiritual practice. The primary difference in tone surrounding self-care tips during the pandemic was that these methods often seemed to be one's only safe option for moving forward while the world ground to a halt around them (Ray 1996, Murray 2015, Lucchetti et al. 2021, Steinert 2021, Teplin 2021).

2 Carl Jung and Other Witches

One of the practices that I observed across social media is shadow work. Particularly on platforms such as TikTok, one would be hard pressed to find experienced members of the community who do not insist that new members devote serious time and energy toward doing shadow work. This practice is a kind of meditation meant to explore what negative energies and upsetting experiences one has been refusing to acknowledge, so they can come to terms with these memories and potentially seek therapy before moving forward in their witchcraft practice. The rationale is that the psyche is part of the human instrument, and the entire instrument is used in every ritual action. Being completely aware of all the cracks and crevices is not only good for spiritual upkeep but also a mark of good mental health; therefore, it is a widely promoted trend within the online pagan community. As we will examine in further detail later, this practice of meditation therapy is extremely Jungian (Murray 2015, von Schnurbein 2016, houseofcraft 2019, witchofthenorse 2019, chris_of_pentacles 2020, Joho & Sung 2020, strega_sarracenia 2020, theglamourwitchla 2020, Lucchetti et al. 2021).

The roots of shadow work are disputed within the online community. This community is made up of those who are active participants within faith-based discussion on public-access internet forums. By its very nature, this community is centralized in urban locations and the global north, which serves to influence the perspective of the majority. The most widely agreed upon origin of shadow work is that the practice combines methods of talk therapy and deep breathing meditation. Talk therapy, which was first implemented in the late 19th century by Dr. Joseph Breuer and Ms. Anna O, and popularized by Dr. Sigmund Freud (Sandhu 2015), is a psychotherapy technique that is often referred to as the ideal model for shadow work. The practitioner is both the therapist and the patient: the present self is the therapist, and the traumatized past self is the patient. Journaling, prayer, and meditative self-reflection are some of the more popular ways in which the present-self and the past-self communicate during these therapeutic events. Those who have gone through extremely traumatic life events often credit their professional licensed therapists as being helpful in their spiritual journey as well. This reinforces how important the maintenance of mental health is within the 21st century pagan community (Ivakhiv 2005, Lepage 2013, Murray 2015, Lucchetti et al. 2021).

Shadow work is often performed under the guidance of a supernatural entity, such as a patron goddess or an ancestor's spirit. Paganism, in its various forms, is a philosophy and a religious expression that prioritizes mental and emotional well-being. Working with a professional therapist is considered good practice in the same way that one would seek outside help for any other endeavor. When members of the pagan community discuss shadow work online, strategies of maintaining and improving mental health go hand in hand with the nurturing of community and everyone's role in the group (Murray 2015, Duda 2021). Often, the professional therapist is referred to as being adjacent to these pagan communities, even though the therapist's own religious views are rarely known. These concepts all refer to reconstructing archetypical theories of community-building, in which everyone contributed toward the future of the group by taking on domestic tasks as required. For many pagans who make this a central point in their group structure, there is a strong Jungian element of predestination to justify why they choose one task over another (Lepage 2013, Murray 2015, von Schnurbein 2016). One survey[1] participant described themselves as having "always been an organized person, an early riser," which was a trait they claimed was evident in other blood relations. This was a driving reason why they put themselves in charge of learning to cook and having breakfast ready for everyone else and factored into why their friends and housemates referred to them as a paternal figure within their circle. This early-rising survey participant was several months into their shadow work at the time of the study, and they noted that they attempted to do so, wherever possible, in a wooded location, as they felt that it brought them closer to their Sámi heritage (Teplin 2021).

Why is such a thorough examination of the darkest crevasses of the self a requirement for the 21st-century witch? Done for at least a few minutes of meditation a day, every day, for months at a time, this is the spiritual construction period meant to fine tune the instrument that is intended to make supernatural changes to the interconnected world around them. When considering how shadow work functions as a foundation of technique in 21st-century witchcraft, it is easier to step back and examine the whole practice. Witcraft can be a philosophy as much as it can be a religion, which is why its practices go hand in hand with so many other religious beliefs. Moreover, the philosophy of using one's own power to get tasks done through knowledge of the natural as well as the supernatural gives witchcraft staying power and has allowed it, in some form, to exist for as long as it has. In relation to our overarching point, the ability to process past trauma during a period of rapid and potentially traumatic change is an effective way to care for oneself. Simply put, confronting the shadow self is self-care.

3 The Private Curation of the Spirit

One of the most common doctrines of witchcraft among current online discourse is that your psychological state will have a direct impact on what you are creating. Being present during a task is a technique common to self-help gurus, hippies, and pagans in this regard. Among those who were surveyed, more than half expressed ideas of how mentorship from spirits, gods, and members of the community (deceased or otherwise) would assist in controlling emotional states during ritual work. The stresses of performing mundane tasks during a global pandemic, whether or not in isolation, can and should be considered within the context of their spiritual impact as much as their psychological impact.

The kitchen is, for many cultures, thought to be the center of home life. As people were restricted to their homes for varying lengths of time during the pandemic, the kitchen gained further importance as the home became the only place people could be at. However, for those who use activities within the home to express their faith, the kitchen is a key ritual space. In this case, the term "kitchen witch" generally denotes someone who does ritual work within the context of food production. Among those surveyed, 8% actively used activities in the kitchen in the practice of their faith, and 2% of those participants were among the 6% who recalled having an older relative that used the kitchen for a similar ritual practice (Teplin 2021). Often, domestic activities that play a ritualistic role are repetitive and function in the same way that rosaries do within Catholic prayer practices. Kneading bread, stirring a pot, and cleaning dishes are all repetitive, careful motions, which are a convenient opportunity for a pagan to invoke an ancestor, relevant deity, or patron saint (Ginzburg 1992, Magliocco 2004, Murray 2007, Stark 2007). Prayers, good intentions, and other supernatural components can be worked into the mixture along with the physical ingredients. Moreover, this central space can be an area of depositing offerings.

Baked goods and foods are a common part of ritual events, falling into one of two categories that are not always mutually exclusive: offerings and feasts. The creation of these materials does allow for a more personal involvement in ritual practices than would be possible from purchasing offerings. It is this hands-on element, preparing materials throughout the day and bringing one's practice into mundane activities, that many survey participants (30% of those who had completed the survey in full) noted was a positive reaffirmation of their faith. None of these participants had a permanent altar within the kitchen space, and 12% of participants indicated setting up a temporary altar in the kitchen space either for a holiday event or specific ritual activity. As there were numerous supply chain issues during the pandemic, increasing numbers of pagans explored means of self-production, evident in both the responses to the study as well as the topics of posts found on social media. This trend was not found only in the kitchen, but in other domestic activities as well.

The garden has historically been a space tied to the kitchen, and during quarantine, a glut of articles appeared online to assist people in growing vegetables during their increased time at home. Of the 8% of people within the study who identified the kitchen as their primary ritual space, more than half were also among the 14% of participants who said they did a significant amount of ritual practice outdoors involving plant matter. In practice, this is very similar to "kitchen witchcraft," in that the physical labor of caring for plants in the garden was a meditative act that channeled the intentions of the practitioner. The plants were largely herbal or vegetable in nature; they were grown to be used in teas, food, and other consumables. Of the study participants, 4% had an altar within their gardens for ritual work (Teplin 2021).

Cooking and gardening initially appear to be at odds with the parameters for the non-activities of self-care laid out at the beginning of this chapter. However, these chores are done for personal gain, both in the spiritual and practical sense, which feeds back into the core ideal of putting oneself first to alleviate a stressful situation. Moreover, the repetitive nature of these domestic activities creates a space for meditation that is often touted as beneficial among self-care advocates. Those in this study who associated garden spaces with the sacred drew most of their inspirations from the regenerative properties of nature, citing reasons such as seeing the progress of growth in plant life, the meditative nature of repetitive labor, and the ability to connect with the planet on a personal level by working in a garden. Regaining a sense of growth and progress during the pandemic was cited as being a key component in maintaining hope and composure by multiple members of this study.

Another mundane activity that was sacralized among members of this study that adheres to the more epicurean aspects of the self-care movement was water-based ritual work. For the 8% of surveyed participants who primarily did rituals that focused on water, the bathtub was where most of their ritual work took place during the pandemic. Prior to this, for half of these participants, the bathtub was not the primary ritual space, as they tried to use outdoor bodies of water (such as lakes) wherever possible. Ritual bathing, in general, is a different meditative format than those tied to domestic activities. Within the kitchen and the garden, a repetitive, practical task is imbued with ritual meaning, and the faith and intentions of the practitioner make the end product somehow special and magical. With ritual bathing, the practitioners themselves are becoming worked on and changed by their environment through meditation, scrubbing, prayer, and the use of religious consumables (candles, incense, and a variety of talisman objects).

Ritual washing gains a new depth of meaning when performed during isolation caused by a pandemic, and ideas of cleansing on a spiritual level were not usually separated from the task of sanitizing as a protective measure against COVID-19. Sanitizing a space in a ritual sense requires the confidence that one can control and understand, to some degree, what one is cleansing. Particularly in the early days of the pandemic, when ideas of how the virus spread were still being tested, the act of cleansing itself could potentially reinvigorate anxieties of contamination. This speaks to the feedback loop of anxiety created by current events and isolation that many members of the study were contending with, a sentiment which was echoed in online forums (Saltzman 2020, Loades et al. 2020, Lucchetti 2021).

4 The Public Curation of the Community

Within 21st-century pagan faith groups[2] the internet was treated more of a resource guide than as a space for ritual interaction. However, this does not indicate a lack of noticeable change in internet use during the pandemic. The open-discourse nature of the evolving theology surrounding contemporary paganism meant that, with more practitioners online, there was an increase in discussion surrounding practices, hereditary crafts, cultural appropriation, and what it means when ritual work lives on the internet. Moreover, practices that shared space with more mainstream ideas of reducing stress and improving one's life could be under scrutiny more easily in an open forum. A kitchen witch might cite a juice cleanse as a great way to get their health on track, creating one avenue by which health and occult communities interchange information. Most online communities have their own forms of self-policing, and this exchange of membership often leads to participants from one community scrutinizing the methods and beliefs of another (Ray 1996, Carrier et al. 2015, Saunders 2020).

Theory of practice is actively developing within pagan communities online as issues arise within public forums. While there is an element of seniority within these communities—a seniority of experience, not in age—it must be noted that there is a general lack of hierarchy within these debates. In the pagan community at large, an effort is made to be egalitarian in group activities as much as in theological debate (Ivakhiv 2005, Puryear 2006, von Schnurbein 2016). This has created an environment in which the examination of the *whys* of ritual practice is as important and as commonly discussed as the *hows*. The shift to digital forums helps to facilitate this discussion, as does the way that social media quickly shifted the community from local to global. This happened gradually and haphazardly over the course of 40 years: the use of mail-order subscriptions, yearly conventions, and limited in-person vetting of closely knit groups gave way to an omnipresent stream of global contact (Magliocco 2004, Stark 2007, Harvey 2009, Lepage 2013, Stager 2015, von Schnurbein 2016).

Within the self-help community, many ideas and methods can trace their origins and reputation back to daytime television, where practices are less subject to scientific rigor and more reliant on the gift of gab (Favazza & Conterio 1988, Ray 1996, Quail et al. 2005, Stager 2015). Now that the self-help community has moved to online spaces, discussions are dominated by personal anecdotes—just as in many discussions on personal ritual—with the topics instead being focused on medicine and science. It is when one falls into the trap of using a religious ritual to de-stress in one forum and then claiming medical benefits from that same ritual in another forum that contention between the two parties starts to arise. During the pandemic, isolation measures led to a rise in participation on social justice forums and social justice demonstrations, as well as in the spreading of information about where and how these injustices were taking place (Saunders 2020, Steinert 2021, Greene et al. 2022). Lockdown allowed people the time to be exposed to an outside perspective and thereby become educated on relevant subjects. Members of the self-help and witchcraft communities who were in online spaces during this time were observed bonding over shared ideals (e.g., self-actualization, the rejuvenating power of nature, health benefits from home-grown food) and clashing over difference in practice (e.g., innate feminine power vs. universal power, restrictive dieting, leaving offerings). For those who openly practiced paganism or witchcraft and touted themselves as being a part of the self-help movement, there were a few key practices that were repeatedly observed as being shared, such as meditation or a specific diet.

Ritual feasting, pilgrimage, offerings, and prayer are universal features of religious expression. An examination of the discussions occurring online as well as the thoughts on the matter among the participants of the study revealed that prayer and pilgrimage were more likely to be forms of expression that were done solo and constructed privately by the individual, though they would be informed by outside information. Ritual feasting and situations in which food and drink were shared often followed models and guidelines suggested by other members of the community, and these events would look similar across different groups (Magliocco 2001, Eliferova 2008, Murray 2015, Lucchetti 2021). Offerings also followed guidelines: while pilgrimage, feasts, and offerings all leaned heavily on the archeological record of how these forms of religious expression existed in the past, what offerings to leave on which altar and when is the most agreed-upon information passed around in these spaces (Magliocco 2001, Puryear 2006, Eliferova 2008, Stager 2015). The nature of manufactured knowledge and what is and isn't worthy information in the founding of religious practice can be a whole book unto itself. In practice, information on preferred offerings is often gathered through websites created by practitioners, which refer to each other in a rabbit warren of translations of the Norse Eddahs and Gerald Gardner tracts. The construction of all belief systems, historically speaking, is a similar game of telephone. What this construction borne of textural reinterpretation suggests is that the future of New Age religious belief systems is going to look markedly different as real-time communication helps them to evolve into a potentially more universal set of neo-pagan beliefs.

Examining how much perceived freedom to alter ritual patterns a 21st-century pagan has brings up to what degree each practice is reconstructionist (i.e., taking an approach where ancient faith systems are interpreted from the standpoint of a practitioner with a modern thought system) or orthodox (i.e., one that attempts to function theoretically from the standpoint of those who had constructed the ancient faith systems in question). Meditation was an overwhelmingly common practice and employed for a myriad of purposes. During the pandemic, meditation was utilized, among other reasons, to create more purposeful personal habits, as a means to prayer, and to regain control of one's emotional state (houseofcraft 2019, witchofthenorse 2020, Duda 2021, Lucchetti 2021, Teplin 2021).

The wide varieties of supernatural world-systems encompassed by the term *contemporary paganism* have a common thread: the idea that spiritual guidance could be sought from members of similar faiths who have died. Another common belief was that the afterlife was either non-existent or not something the living should be too concerned with. Of the survey's participants, 74% believe in some form of communication between the living and their ancestors, 42% do not feel the need to ascribe to a firm philosophy on the afterlife, and 36% overlap in holding both beliefs simultaneously (Teplin 2021). As so many contemporary pagan communities are becoming multi-generational, what do these prevalent ideas mean for relationships with death and family memorials on a personal level? This question, unfortunately, must be answered by future research. However, we can start to examine what neo-pagan ideas surrounding death and the afterlife look like within the context of discussions surrounding death in the pandemic.

The eminent presence of death and concerns surrounding one's own health came to the fore for many religious groups in 2020, and the pagan community was no exception. These concerns were often discussed in public forums, where pagans tried to find a community in which to garner support and comfort during times of emotional and literal isolation (Howick & Rees 2017, Loades et al. 2020, Saltzman et al. 2020, Steinert 2021). These discussions occurred more frequently on social media sites that were text-based as well as hidden from the general public (e.g., FaceBook, Reddit, and Discord servers), rather than those which were video-based (e.g., TikTok and Twitch). This anxiety is aside from the more widespread topics of loneliness in quarantine, or of feelings of being isolated at home due to having no other members of their faith to interact with, or to needing to hide their beliefs and practices from those they live with (witchofthenorse 2019, Khademi et al 2020, strega_sarracenia 2020, Lucchetti 2021, Loades et al. 2020). The discussions that focus specifically on pandemic-related stress often include how ritual practice and shadow work can be adapted to address fears of sickness and death. These same conversations would inform ideas of how to approach the afterlife, especially as relatives of those who were in these forums succumbed to COVID-19 (Khademi et al. 2020, Saltzman et al. 2020, Lucchetti 2021). There were little to no changes observed in which gods were being worshipped, nor in the specific ritual processes. Most often, the specific words were what was altered during regular religious activity, or a new item with closer connections to good health was swapped in during normal ritual practice.

5 Whitewashing and Commodity Culture

I would now like to comment on that big asterisk at the beginning of this chapter. A lot of nuances can be expected to be lost along the way when discussing such complex topics as the ways in which supernatural forces interact and our own emotional and mental health. This issue increases exponentially when these ideas are being boiled down to their most easily digestible and basic parts to be disseminated to a wider audience, whether to increase awareness about a practice, invite participation to a holiday, or to sell something. The biggest problems lie in the question of who is the common denominator being catered to. The 21st-century witchcraft community emphasizes a knowledge of practice. This is easily done through the ease at which not only information is accessed, but at which people from the marginalized cultures (where these ritual practices can be traced back to) can be accessed. The specifics of ritual practices change over time and are often marked with references back to their originating culture. This is seen, for example, in the arrangement of specific feathers on the clothing worn during Indigenous American dances. A cornerstone of debate in these online spaces was how to change the way people had been approaching closed practices. In online occult spaces and beyond, there has been a prevalent theme that peoples whose practices had been subject to ridicule and erasure should not have to see those same practices worn as a costume by people from outside their communities.

We have already examined the idea of how and where the commodification of religious paraphernalia occurs earlier in this chapter. Within the issue of commercialization is the problem of the impact made by the procurement of ritual materials, such as eagle feathers or white sage, and this is a heated topic of debate within the pagan community today. This debate had a further dimension added in 2020. During the pandemic, the logistics of production were hugely impacted, making the transportation of goods wildly unpredictable. Ritual that is built on traditions of imitation without an understanding of the specific reasoning behind each action results in religious events being disrupted by a lack of one specific type of dried herb or a bowl made out of a certain material.

Several issues that have been brought up in this chapter can be traced back to one idea: the "footprint" of one's spiritual practice. This includes the negative impact one makes on contributing to environmental damage by using specific materials for ritual, of burning out oneself and those around them by not working through past trauma in a healthy way, and by commandeering sacred practices from other cultures, whether knowingly or not. In an interconnected and global world, it is impossible not to create damage with one's footprint, no matter how lightly one treads.

6 Conclusions

Through discourse and debate, 21st-century witches have used online tools to ensure a healthy and supportive community with generally accessible information. At the same time, the specific ideas of how the supernatural operates can vary wildly between individual practitioners, despite a similarity in the material aspects of religious expression. At the core of what it means to define witchcraft in the 21st century is to examine materialism, the pedigree of faith systems, one's own emotional health, and the impact of one's "footprint." All of these are means to self-empowerment. This supernatural perspective on self-care is the reason why many who practice witchcraft combine it as a philosophical outlook with a religious practice or as an atheist.

The evolving relationship with the sacred and the supernatural is being increasingly influenced by how we interact with the mundane and tangible. In practical terms, this is evidenced by how we adapt our ritual patterns: modern hurdles require modern solutions, and theological debate has allowed for both a wider cast of speakers and a more nuanced series of topics through the internet. Within the context of 21st-century paganism, we must review these themes through the lens of self-empowerment and alternate, often more direct forms of finding spiritual fulfillment.

Notes

1 To note: the survey described within this chapter refers to the survey used in the data collection for the MA thesis "God is My Quarantine Buddy." This survey was a series of open-answer questions about practice, accompanied by some multiple choice questions about self-identification. Each participant was a member of a different meeting group (such as a coven or kindred), and meeting groups from multiple faiths were surveyed. These faiths included Asatru, Kemetism, Wicca, Celtic Druidry, and others.

2 Pagan faith groups here refers to those who are active within these online communal spaces. The majority of these are of younger generations and from the global north, thereby there is a noticeable majority who are Wicca, Asatru, or claim a faith based in traditions stemming from northern Europe. In these groups, a number claimed to be simultaneously agnostic or atheist. There were smaller yet significant groups that promoted discussion focused on Kemetism and Voudoo, as well as groups that promoted the blending of Indigenous American faith systems with other practices. The smallest represented group was that of pre-Josian Judaism.

Works Cited

Burke, Kellie, "The Neuroscience Behind Retail Therapy," (2018) All Regis University Theses. 864. https://epublications.regis.edu/theses/864.

Carrier, L. Mark, et al., "Virtual Empathy: Positive and Negative Impacts of Going Online upon Empathy in Young Adults," *Computers in Human Behavior* 52 (2015): 39–48.

chris_of_pentacles (2020) TikTok. Retrieved from http://www.tiktok.com.

Duda, Viktória G., "From Individual to Collective Shadow Work in Past Life Regression Therapy," Paper Presented to the *Global Integral Awakens Conference*, Hungary, 2021. http://www.viktoriaduda.com/uploads/1/7/0/0/17001902/shadow_in_regression_therapy.pdf.

Eliferova, Maria, "Public and Non-Public Space in Anglo-Saxon and Norse Culture," *Cultural Perspectives-Journal for Literary and British Cultural Studies in Romania* 13 (2008): 13–20.

Favazza, Armando R., and Karen Conterio, "The Plight of Chronic Self-Mutilators," *Community Mental Health Journal* 24.1 (1988): 22–30.

Ginzburg, Carlo, *The Night Battles: Witchcraft and Agrarian Cults in the Sixteenth and Seventeenth Centuries* (trans. by John & Anne Tedeschi), Baltimore, MD: Johns Hopkins University Press, 1992.

Greene, Amanda K., et al. "'An Immaculate Keeper of My Social Media Feed': Social Media Usage in Body Justice Communities during the COVID-19 Pandemic," *Social Media+ Society* 8.1 (2022): 20563051221077024.

Harvey, Graham, "Animist Paganism," in *Handbook of Contemporary Paganism*, edited by Murphy Pizza and James Lewis, Leiden: Brill, 2009, 393–412.

houseofcraft (2019–2020) TikTok. Retrieved from http://www.tiktok.com.

Howick, Jeremy, and S. Rees, "Overthrowing Barriers to Empathy in Healthcare: Empathy in the Age of the Internet," *Journal of the Royal Society of Medicine* 110.9 (2017): 352–357.

Ivakhiv, Adrian, "Have We (N)ever Been Natural? Have We (N)ever Been Ethnic? The 'Amodernism' of Slavic Neo-Paganism," Paper Read at the American Academy of Religion Annual Meeting in Philadelphia, 2005 (unpublished).

Joho, Jess, and Sung, Morgan, "How to Be a Witch without Stealing Other People's Cultures," *Mashable*, https://mashable.com/article/witchtok-problematic-witch-cultural-appropriation/ Oct 31 2020.

Kang, Minjeong, and Kim KP Johnson, "Retail Therapy: Scale Development," *Clothing and Textiles Research Journal* 29.1 (2011): 3–19.

Khademi, Fatemeh, Siamak Moayedi, and Mohamad Golitaleb, "The COVID-19 Pandemic and Death Anxiety in the Elderly," *International Journal of Mental Health Nursing* 30.1 (2020): 346–349.

Lee, Jihyun, and Yuri Lee, "Does Online Shopping Make Consumers Feel Better? Exploring Online Retail Therapy Effects on Consumers' Attitudes towards Online Shopping Malls," *Asia Pacific Journal of Marketing and Logistics* 31 (2019): 464–479.

Lepage, Martin, "A Lokian Family: Queer and Pagan Agency in Montreal," *The Pomegranate* 15.1–2 (2013): 79–101.

Loades, Maria Elizabeth, et al., "Rapid Systematic Review: The Impact of Social Isolation and Loneliness on the Mental Health of Children and Adolescents in the Context of COVID-19," *Journal of the American Academy of Child & Adolescent Psychiatry* 59.11 (2020): 1218–1239.

Lucchetti, Giancarlo, et al., "Spirituality, Religiosity and the Mental Health Consequences of Social Isolation during Covid-19 Pandemic," *The International Journal of Social Psychiatry* 67.6 (2021): 672.

Magliocco, Sabina, *Neo-Pagan Sacred Art and Altars: Making Things Whole*, Jackson: University of Mississippi Press, 2001.

Magliocco, Sabina, *Witching Culture: Folklore and Neo-Paganism in America*, Philadelphia: University of Pennsylvania Press, 2004.

Magnell, Ola, and Elisabeth Iregren, "Veitstu hvé blóta skal? The old Norse blót in the light of osteological remains from Frösö church, Jämtland, Sweden," *Current Swedish Archaeology* 18.1 (2010): 223–250.
Murray, Margaret Alice, *The Witch-Cult in Western Europe*, Filiquarian Publishing, LLC, 2007 [public domain document].
Murray, Tom, "Contemplative Dialogue Practices: An Inquiry into Deep Interiority, Shadow Work, and Insight," *Integral Leadership Review; Featured Article* (2015) http://integralleadershipreview.com/13382-819-contemplative-dialogue-practices-an-inquiry-into-deep-interiority-shadow-work-and-insight/.
Puryear, Mark, *The Nature of Ásatrú: An Overview of the Ideals and Philosophy of the Indigenous Religion of Northern Europe*, Bloomington, IN: iUniverse Publishing, (2006).
Quail, Christine M., Kathalene A. Razzano, and Loubna H. Skalli, *Vulture Culture: The Politics and Pedagogy of Daytime Television Talk Shows*, New York, NY: Peter Lang, Inc. Publishing, 2005.
Ray, George B., *Communication and Disenfranchisement: Social Health Issues and Implications* Routledge, (1996) eISBN 9780203812020.
Rodriguez, Jesus Fernando Guerrero, *Old Norse Drinking Culture*. Diss. York: University of York, 2007.
Sandhu, Pavi, *Step Aside, Freud: Josef Breuer Is the True Father of Modern Psychotherapy, Scientific American, Mind Guest Blog*, (2015) https://blogs.scientificamerican.com/mind-guest-blog/step-aside-freud-josef-breuer-is-the-true-father-of-modern-psychotherapy/.
Saltzman, Leia Y., Tonya Cross Hansel, and Patrick S. Bordnick, "Loneliness, Isolation, and Social Support Factors in Post-COVID-19 Mental Health," *Psychological Trauma: Theory, Research, Practice, and Policy* 12.S1 (2020): 55–57.
Saunders, Fenella, "Quarantine Stories," *American Scientist* 108.5 (2020): 258–259.
von Schnurbein, Stefanie, "Creating the Paradigm: Historical Preconditions of Modern Asatru," *Norse Revival*, Leiden: Brill, 2016.
Stager, Brad, "Considering Mailer in the Post-Aquarian Age," *The Mailer Review* 9.1 (2015): 241–245.
Stark, Rodney, *Discovering God: The Origins of the Great Religions and the Evolution of Belief*, New York, NY: Harper Collins, 2007.
Steinert, Steffen, "Corona and Value Change: The Role of Social Media and Emotional Contagion," *Ethics and Information Technology* 23.1 (2021): 59–68.
strega_sarracenia (2020) TikTok. Retrieved from http://www.tiktok.com.
Teplin, Milo-Rhys K., *God Is My Quarantine Buddy: Debates in Ritual Practice Among North American Pagans in 2020*, Master's Thesis, University of Houston, Anthropology Department, Aug 2021 https://uh-ir.tdl.org/handle/10657/8339.
theglamourwitchla (2020) TikTok. Retrieved from http://www.tiktok.com.
witchofthenorse (2019) TikTok. Retrieved from http://tiktok.com.
Yang, Alan, "Pawnee Rangers" Parks and Rec, Created by Greg Daniels & Michael Schur, Season 4, Episode 4, National Broadcasting Company (NBC), Oct 13th 2011.

12 Pedagogy of Death in the Era of #Coronachaos

Keith E. McNeal

Death is a magical mirror for self and society, as our responses to it are always about life as well. Philosopher Herbert Fingarette (1996) observes that death is without subjective meaning except for how we experience it vicariously through others as well as deal with loss and change: "I, this consciousness, will never know death first hand. In the end, I'm invulnerable. From the subjective point of view my deepest wish is guaranteed—I am immune to death" (p. 6). He reaches this position through a secular route as compared to the usual theological one. Our commonsense response to death obscures an existential truth: one's death will not be an event in one's own life. Thus, our relationship with death is always about our relationship to life and is mediated by society, culture, and experience. It is a mirror for collective reflection and debate.

Put anthropologically, death operates as a screen for socio-symbolic projection of and for human feeling, thought, and imagination for a peculiar primate species that became bipedal, began using increasingly complex tools, developed a high brain-body ratio, and captured fire, the synergistic effects of all of which gave rise to the capacity for symbolic cognition underwriting full-blown language and an astonishing complexification of consciousness, levels of self-awareness and intersubjectivity, and forms of collective behavior. When we became "human" and what counts as "culture" are open to discussion and debate, but we know is that *Homo sapiens* made the morphological transition from "archaic" to "modern" around two hundred thousand years ago and spread outside of Africa, as several earlier species of Homo had, and eventually outcompeted all other hominins. The central plotline here concerns the deepening and complexifying evolution of sociocultural behavior predicated upon intersubjective symbolic cognition and its kaleidoscopic affordances: creativity and imagination, along with temporal consciousness about past and future, all parsed by the extraordinarily variable syntax, grammar, and lexicon of language. Yet since spoken language quickly vanishes into thin air, the earliest archeological signs of symbolic cognition are colored pigments made from natural materials for marking, decorating, and accessorizing. This dawning of our aesthetic impulse arose less than a hundred thousand years ago, followed by the emergence of rock

DOI: 10.4324/b22930-15

and cave art alongside the *earliest evidence for burial and mortuary ritualization* (Kelly 2016). How utterly consequential that the transformative cultural praxis of death is so central within the horizon of possibility afforded by the capacity for symbolic cognition?

This essay is part of a larger work contemplating death, sociality, and ritual from a comparative perspective in the era of what I dub #Coronachaos. I have been working on the historical anthropology of Indo-Caribbean death and mortuary ritual for some time now (McNeal 2018, 2023). This, combined with long-term engagement with the anthropology of religion, inspired me to develop a new course on the Anthropology of Death and Mortuary Ritual that I taught in Fall 2020 at the University of Houston, commencing six months into the pandemic—yet incubated and planned before any sign of COVID-19. Like most of my colleagues, I had to adapt the course to teaching online for the first time under the excruciatingly complex conditions imposed by the global pandemic. COVID-19 then took my grandmother, which I shared with my students by anthropologizing my family's experience as a live case study. My students pursued a host of fascinating and revelatory research projects on death and mortuary ritual within the local pandemic. I consider my own pandemic-prompted spirituality as well as the poignant irony of finding more community with my students online than with my family living in another state, who could not congregate to commemorate and ritualize my grandmother's passing. And I conclude by querying some of death's deeper history and possible futures in light of COVID-19's status as an Anthropocenic disease, a tiny piece of inert RNA that became a global monster.

Enter #Coronachaos

There is no question that teaching the anthropology of death and mortuary rituals benefited immensely in pedagogical terms from doing so less than six months into an epic global pandemic. This is a point of great poignant irony. The topic was live, overbearing, and all around, affecting everyone in countless ways, inflicting enormous pain and suffering, and super-complicating already complicated lives as the world stumbled and fumbled its way forward. I cannot recall exactly when I started speaking about #Coronachaos, with the hashtag mimed in the air, 2nd-and-3rd-fingers-perpendicularly-across-the-other-two. But one day it popped into my head and jumped out of my mouth, quickly taking hold in my conversations with others. People found it poignantly welcome, the hashtag signifying how deeply mediated the pandemic was through burgeoning social media and proliferating new virtual platforms, smartphone applications, and recursive processes of digitalization controlled and surveilled by media corporations and the nation-states that caretake and depend upon them. The term points toward the whole huge, astonishing, vertiginous mess that was the advent of SARS-2-COVID-19—a zoonotic-Anthropogenic disease—on the global stage and the reverberating effects it had and continues to have on our lives, our social relations, our future. #Coronachaos not only implicates the disease itself but also the multifarious implications and consequences resulting from COVID-19. I like to think that the term belongs in the *ecotopian lexicon* curated by Schneider-Mayerson and Bellamy (2019).

Death, cosmology, and mortuary ritualization are interconnected. COVID-19 dramatized and raised the stakes of the game in an epic new way on the global stage. #Coronachaos threatened and diminished lives and livelihoods while disrupting and reshaping death, grief, corpse disposal, patterns of ritualization, and memorialization around the world. COVID-19 strained and overwhelmed infrastructure and resources. We witnessed overflowing morgues, crematoria running non-stop, and mass burials. Public health restrictions and social-distancing regulations impeded methods of ritualizing the dead, restricted funerals, and limited cremations and cemetery visitations. The abundance of caution that came to organize our lives echoed other plagues—HIV/AIDS, SARS, H1N1, Ebola, to cite some of the most recent—yet this got lost within the swirling #Coronachaos. The implications of these changes and transformations are still emerging, but popular media, news commentary, political discourse, and other voices began pointing to them. Yet people and communities around the world responded to COVID-19 with great creative energies, generating new cultural practices and novel deployments of technology.

We had to relearn how to live and die during the pandemic—not always for the first time, of course (the latter a conceit of privileged Global Northernfolk), but under astonishing new conditions of distancing and lockdown. Many died, and grieved, alone. It was a waking nightmare for the living, yet let us not forget how profoundly distressing it was for those dying as well. Losing recourse to ready-made forms of family, community, ritual, and religion in the face of omnipresent death was exquisitely painful and challenging for everyone, across faith traditions and class divisions throughout the world. Most countries not only banned large gatherings but also prohibited travel, further complicating everything—prompting adaptations, compromise solutions and added #Coronachaos, including outright conflict between mourners and authorities as well as instances of flagrant disobedience of public-health restrictions. Examples include ultra-Orthodox Jewish funerals in New York City (Felter et al. 2020) and ancestralist-oriented Bamileke "body snatching" in Cameroon (Ngade 2021).

In the midst of all the talk of radical newness, however, it is anthropologically relevant to note a few exceptional traditions relatively unaffected by the pandemic, such as "sky burials" (corpse disposal by vulture consummation) among Parsis and Buddhists in India, for example (Frayer et al. 2020), as well as traditions revived by the pandemic, such as Scottish recuperation of processional bowing along public funerary routes from yesteryear (Felter et al. 2020). The world adapted, compromised, and innovated. It went even more deeply online, however haphazardly and ambivalently. Jews held virtual Shiva. Han Chinese tomb-sweeping went online. The Holy Spirit was live-streamed. Some Sierra Leoneans defaulted to recent socially distanced modes of funerary praxis, carrying the legacy of civil war in the 1990s and still in living collective memory. Meanwhile, Brazilian gravediggers—even more necessary during a pandemic—faced increased prejudice (Mural 2020). Americans of color faced the intensified perils of life and death while virtually attending George Floyd's funeral in Houston and navigating the changing local and national terrain of #BLM (PBS 2020; Bloomfield 2021). Floyd was from Houston, indeed Third Ward, the very area in which the University of Houston sits, expands, and gentrifies. We spoke about all of this in class online while dispersed throughout the fourth largest city in the USA by population and largest in terms of total area. University of Houston's undergraduate population is considered to be the most diverse in the country given Houston's own mega-diversity vis-à-vis national and international parameters (Klineberg 2020).

Granny Kay and a Spiritual Interlude

The pandemic got very personal, very quickly. My then-90-year-old maternal grandmother, whom we called Granny Kay (short for Katherine), was alive and well enough going into the pandemic. She lived down the hall from my step grandmother (herself then 95 years old) in an assisted-care facility in Tulsa, Oklahoma, where they not only had each other, but also my mom, stepdad, sister, stepsister, and all their families who were able to visit and make the rounds. Lockdown hit Granny Kay less harshly than it did my step grandmother since Mamadottie—as we call her (Dottie from Dorothy)—is the more social of the two. Granny Kay was sociable too but didn't need as much social contact, already spending more time alone in her little apartment than did Mamadottie even before the pandemic descended, consigning them to their rooms. One small mercy was that the facility is a single-floor residential complex with each unit having windows where visitors could come up on the lawn to visit and shout through the window in conversation.

Yet our Granny Kay fell in early October, breaking her arm and injuring her hip. She was taken—alone—by ambulance to the hospital, where she underwent reconstructive surgery and spent several days recovering. Fortunately, my sister was a nurse working in the same hospital, so she was able to visit Granny Kay in clinical-grade protective gear while on shift and give her reassurance and love from the family, even FaceTiming on her phone so we could see Granny Kay and her us. But she was otherwise alone, except for contact with clinical staff. Then she was relocated—again, all alone—to a physical-therapy facility for the elderly and those in need of complete assistance due to injuries, surgeries, and disabilities. That facility was operating under highly restricted conditions, of course, yet even so, it is where Granny Kay somehow contracted COVID-19 after entering the facility. We will never exactly know how she got the novel coronavirus, but presumably from one of the people working there. Had she not fallen and hurt herself, Granny Kay would have never entered this rollercoaster ride that put her on a collision course with COVID-19.

A few days after the diagnosis, I packed up my car to drive nine hours north to visit her. We couldn't take anything for granted. I was teaching online anyway, so spending a week with family in Oklahoma and visiting Granny Kay, again from the lawn through her room window since this facility was also—most fortunately—a single-story complex. We were all trying not to, but quietly fearing the worst. I visited her twice daily, once in the mornings and again in the afternoons. She was not always awake, and when she was, she was not always fully cognizant. Though sometimes she was alert, quietly sitting in her wheelchair by the window, looking out. She was very weak and frail by that point and we could barely understand her trying to speak through the window. It felt awkward and harsh yelling through the window so that she could hear us, but this was the only option except for when an attendant was present and could answer her phone and hold it up to her ear for her to hear us speaking via phone, looking at each other from each side of the window. She was alone inside, and there was nothing we could do except show up and offer her love in a clumsy game of charades through the window. Every visit was heartbreaking.

After a week, I drove back to Houston, feeling helpless and heartbroken. A mere nine days after bidding her goodbye at her room window, at 12.20 am on Saturday, October 17, Granny Kay died in her sleep. My mom called around 7.30 am that morning with the news. When I heard the phone buzzing on my bedside table, I immediately knew what it was, since everyone knows I am not a morning person and should never call early. COVID-19 had taken my own grandmother, stealing her from us prematurely. Making matters worse, there was no funeral because they were still disallowed. I had been cooped up in my place in Houston during the lockdown, and now I was still cooped up, sitting with this tragedy alone at home. The phone barely rang. Literally, nothing happened.

Granny Kay had been an organ donor, but her COVID-19-positive body was not accepted for donation. There was a backlog of corpses for cremation due to the pandemic, so it was two and a half months before she was cremated, and then another month and a half before her ashes were available. My mom texted a photo of the urn with Granny Kay's remains on the table behind her sofa. Given that my 75-year-old stepfather was then undergoing chemotherapy treatment for lymphoma, the family decided—not without conflict or debate (#MoreCoronachaos)—not to gather for Thanksgiving or Christmas that year and put him or anyone else at any further health risk. I drove up to see my mother for her birthday in March 2021, when I was able to lay my hands on the urn with Granny's ashes inside. Then, on Mother's Day in May, my mom, her siblings, and their spouses visited central Oklahoma for a highly delayed, eight-person interment ceremony, burying my grandmother's remains in the ground next to her second husband, my step grandfather, who had died from cancer years before and had burial rights in a military cemetery because of his service in the Marines during the Korean War. Only when I visited again later in the year was I able to visit the cemetery myself and pay my respects, a full ten months after her death and without any form of ritualization marking the occasion. I stood next to her gravesite, watching a groundskeeper mow the grass nearby.

But I need to backtrack here in order to finish telling this part of the story. Ever since my grandmother was diagnosed with COVID-19, I had been intending to sit down and chant the *Liberation From Sorrow: Praises and Requests to the Twenty-One Tārās*, a Vajrayana Buddhist liturgical prayer that invokes the 21 forms of Tārā—a Wisdom Buddha, often called the Female Buddha or the Mother of Liberation. I had been given the root mantra for Green Tārā when I was 21 years old in India and had always kept it close to my heart, though my practice of Buddhism has intermittently waxed and waned over the years. Even before the advent of COVID-19, I had been developing a modest practice of meditating at home in front of my altar, but then—like many people—dealing with lockdown and #Coronachaos saw me at home all the time wrestling with my heart-mind amid the socially distanced madness. Thus, my practice had been deepening and developing momentum. I was reading and practicing my Buddhism even more, including online pujas and Zoomed teachings. I had recently gotten my hands on a copy of *Liberation From Sorrow* and come to appreciate it more. Hence, I had been wanting to sit and devote an entire session of chanting this prayer for Granny Kay ever since her diagnosis.

I returned to Houston on Sunday, October 11 and then teaching and all the rest hurtled me through another week. That following Friday night, I finally got a chance to chant the *Liberation From Sorrow*. Sometime after 11 pm, I turned off all the lights in the house and lit a candle on my altar in the back room, where I sat down and proceeded to chant the prayer. *Oh Arya Tārā, please bestow upon us permanent liberation from the suffering of lower rebirth, permanent liberation from the suffering of samsaric birth, and the great liberation of full enlightenment.* I went into it concerned that I might be too tired to sit comfortably for an hour on my meditation pillow and really wanted my session to be comfy and flow since it was on behalf of Granny Kay, who was suffering alone with COVID-19. But it somehow went very well: I felt comfortable and centered and very connected to and focused upon the chant-prayer and its significance for the suffering of sentient beings. I finished and then sat quietly meditating for at least another 20 minutes, the whole time feeling calm, alert, focused. I was glad I had finally gotten the chance to sit for Granny Kay. After finishing, I blew out the candle and slipped into bed.

The next morning at around 7.30 am, my phone rang, and I've already told that part of the story. It was my mom calling to report that Granny Kay had died overnight. What time did she pass, I asked? 12.20 am, she answered. We spoke for a short while, me groggy from being awoken and both of us in shock about Granny's death. Mom had other people to call, so we said we'd speak again later and hung up. I sat up in bed, trying to digest the news. Wait! 12.20 am? Wasn't that when I was meditating for her? In order to figure out my timing, I checked a WhatsApp message I'd sent to one of my best friends about 20 minutes before sitting down to meditate—it was just a few minutes after 11 pm, which meant I would have sat down and started around 11.20 pm, and that I would have just been reaching the end of the chanted prayer at *exactly* the time that Granny Kay died! I was stunned. And so relieved I hadn't put it off until later that weekend.

My meditation had been so comfortable, centered and meaningful, and then to realize that I was at least with Granny Kay in spirit when she passed was incredibly moving for me. It was all I could do in our socially distanced lockdown conditions. I continued to be sad and mad that she had been taken from us prematurely, but I also felt more peaceful and less guilty about it since I had been with her in the only way I could. This experience blew me away. I shared it with a few friends, as well as my mother and sister, yet no one else in the family since they're Southern Baptists and not interested in my spiritual life. This experience greatly buffered the impact of Granny Kay's death for me personally. It felt extraordinarily consequential, giving me something to hold onto. I reported that Granny Kay had passed to my students in our next class online, as they had been getting the blow-by-blow updates along the way and following the evolving plotline. Granny Kay was somewhere between 199,000 and 200,000 in terms of the American death count at that point during the still-accelerating pandemic, a time when a vaccine was still but a wishful fantasy. I continued to update my students as things slowly progressed bureaucratically with the pathology report and death certificate, etc. Yet Granny Kay's ashes arrived after the end of the semester, so they never heard how the story ended.

Student Research

While I was open about the situation with Granny Kay with my students, anthropologizing my family's experience along the way, I did not share what happened the night she died. That somehow felt too intimate and vulnerable. I thought about it and almost told them, but never did. It gives me pause now thinking about why I opted not to tell them the most exquisite part of the story for me spiritually, and now I partly wish I had. My best student in an all-around excellent class was a passionate, studious young man with whom I had already had several scintillating online office-hour conversations about the course and beyond. As we were gearing up for students to pursue their research projects—I offered a group option, but interestingly, no one went for that—Jimmy Nguyen wanted to chat again about researching the effects of the pandemic within local Buddhist communities (he asked that I use his full name here, personal email communication, Oct. 2022). Then he asked if he could interview me as one of his research subjects since he had learned that I am Buddhist in an earlier conversation and my experience the night Granny Kay died came out in the wash. He was moved.

Jimmy explored the intersections of COVID-19 and Buddhist praxis, focusing on Vietnamese Mahāyāna Buddhists like his family. He considered the pivotal significance of death in Buddhist theology and reflected upon his first trip abroad to Vietnam as an early adult in 2018 in which he attended a funeral that surprised him and was critical of, prompting ruminations on the betwixt-and-betweenness of being Vietnamese-American. He also examined the centrality of mortuary praxis in Vietnamese culture, both at "home" and in diaspora, such as the pervasiveness of ancestral altars alongside domestic Buddhist shrines in Vietnamese homes. Jimmy also conducted an ethnography of a small Vietnamese-Buddhist temple in Houston that remained active throughout the pandemic, augmented by interviews with ten Buddhists—eight of Vietnamese descent and two Anglo-Americans, one of whom attended the temple and the other, an anthropology professor, practicing Buddhism at home alone. Vietnamese Buddhism is prominent within the local scene because Houston was one of the main cities to which Vietnamese migrated after the Vietnam War, at the same time that Houston was materializing as the epicenter of the global fossil-fuel industry. There are around 150 Vietnamese Buddhist temples and many thousands of Vietnamese Buddhists in Houston, many of whom resorted to live streaming local services online. Jimmy's research also disclosed how fewer people visiting temples equaled less donations, with consequences for clergy such as the nun he interviewed, who was struggling financially due to declining contributions while continuing to minister to the heightened needs of lay members. He explored the vicissitudes of Vietnamese and Vietnamese-Americans struggling through the pandemic inflected by both Buddhist theology and traditional ancestralism, experiencing #Coronachaos in ways different from other Houstonians. Many intensified their devotions and praxis as a result of pandemic conditions.

Conducting projects on death and mortuary ritual in Houston was very much invigorated and deepened in significance by doing so in the midst of the pandemic. I found students to be more motivated and ambitious than usual. We devoted several sessions to brainstorming and discussing their ideas and interests, allowing them to discuss and offer feedback to one another in conversation with me. It was all poignant, heady, and exciting despite the relentlessly sad situation we were investigating. And I was blown away by their ideas, projects, commitment, and passion for bringing things to fruition. We devoted a marathon session at the end of the term that allowed them to discuss their projects and think about how the materials we had studied throughout the term could be applied to their findings.

One student interviewed ICU nurses working on the frontlines in hospitals, examining the new clinical and emotional challenges of healthcare, the liminality and micropolitics of ventilators, and the new pragmatics of Zooming in hospitals. Another interviewed doctors and physician's assistants about the grueling dynamics of frontline pandemic work, fascinating yet troubling new ambiguities in clinical diagnosis and comorbidities, the phenomenology of COVID-19, and the political economy of healthcare in the USA. Another culled statistical data regarding the operation, logistics, and economics of hospital healthcare in Houston—a major biomedical center in the country—disclosing how the quickly mushrooming emergency conditions were met with a state-wide ban on elective surgical and major medical procedures in order to meet the challenge. However, this also meant that hospitals therefore experienced a decline in revenue, in turn prompting workforce reductions, further undermining overall clinical readiness and effort. The prohibition on elective procedures was suspended in September 2020, generating a slight bump in hospital revenues. Yet many were still afraid to seek medical attention in hospitals unless absolutely critical and the downward economic spiral continued. These data were plotted in a schematic dashboard presenting trends and changes over time which the student shared with the class. Another student—a Mexican-American female veteran of the Iraq War—drew upon her experience of the local VA hospital in order to pursue ethnographic exploration of the temporary emergency facilities erected in the parking lot and inside the hospital, as well as interviewed four veterans about their experience of #Coronachaos, disclosing the ways that veterans were more vulnerable and at higher risk—including for suicide—than the civilian population due to a convergence of factors that preceded yet were exacerbated by COVID-19.

I also had students looking into the mortuary industry. One student was also studying at the Commonwealth Institute of Funeral Services in Houston, which offers training in funeral directing and embalming. We were all surprised and fascinated when she spoke up about this, and she turned out to be a well-placed informant about the rapidly changing logistics of COVID-19 mortalities, autopsy performance, pathology reporting, corpse disposal, pandemic protocols, and so forth throughout the term. Her project reflected on her own experience combined with interviews with a pathologist and a funeral director about the technical scenario and had an especially intriguing section exploring the steep challenges of living up to the Funeral Service Oath and the subtle kinds of bias and paranoia at work within the mortuary industry during the pandemic, in which COVID-19 was handled differently—with less privacy—than other diseases. Another student reconstructed the changing position and guidelines, as well as politics, of the Centers for Disease Control regarding COVID-19, also considering intensifying trends toward cremation prompted by pandemic conditions, with implications for mortuary customs among various religious traditions. Another's investigation of a local funeral home examined the new challenges and pressures faced by the industry, confirming decline in burial accompanied by increasing cremation as well as falling revenue and profits due to the cessation of funerals, which meant the lack of need for embalming and caskets, etc.

Other students focused on issues concerning subjective experience and mental health. One delved into the challenges for mental health and well-being presented by pandemic conditions, including the pros and cons of telemedicine, the lack of connectivity and community incumbent upon social-distancing, and vicissitudes of suicide before and during the pandemic. Another student considered the intensifying dynamics of social media usage during the pandemic and how they played into the swirling cauldron of #Coronachaos. Another approached me privately, divulging that she was having especially difficult mental health problems in lockdown and asked if she could write autobiographically about herself instead, which I agreed to, and she produced a poignant testament to the trials and tribulations of trying to stay sane in the midst of the pandemic. A woman I'd had in several previous classes who characterized herself as coming from a "white trash" background explored the discourses and dynamics of proletarian Anglo-Texan domestic pandemic drama. An African-American woman similarly examined deaths in her family and the disproportionate hardships visited upon Black families dealing with #Coronachaos.

Only a small number of students chose to research the impact of COVID-19 pandemic upon religiosity. One examined her family's Southern Baptist Church and how the denomination was wrestling with discussion and debate—as well as censoring information—regarding the novel coronavirus. Another student from the Gulf Coast just south of Houston documented the microhistory of the Archdiocese of Galveston Island from the outset of pandemic to the present, including the anguished decision to suspend Masses and offer restricted liturgical services, its phased later reopening, the double whammy of #Coronachaos plus loss of religious community, the challenges and consequences of virtual Mass, and the ways the pandemic was especially difficult for the elderly within the community. A Ghanaian-American student explored the fascinating ways that Ghanaians in diaspora had already pre-adapted to the virtualization of funerary praxis and took the challenges in better stride than other communities.

I also had students probing the implications of pandemic for education. An African-American woman I'd had in several classes who lived on campus and worked part-time next door at Texas Southern University—an HBCU adjacent to UH—examined the ways TSU took a more proactive, compassionate, commonwealth approach whereas UH took a more corporate neoliberal approach. She pursued a fascinating comparative microsociology of temperature-taking on both campuses and concluded that "UH just doesn't care." Another student wrote incisively about the pros and cons of coursework and learning online, as well as the deeply poignant paradoxical experience of losing a family member to COVID-19 and having the death fill up the compressed and claustrophobic space of being in lockdown at home while also having no funeral or way of ritualizing the passage together. I pointed out how ironic it is that in his family's case, he was stuck at home surrounded by the shroud of death yet unable to gather together and mark the moment as part of the post-mortem transition, whereas I was stuck at home alone, my family also unable to gather for any funeral or service together, but whereas he was home with talk of the deceased constantly pervading their shared space, I was in my own house surrounded by a profoundly disturbing quiet. Hall of mirrors similarities and differences in our respective experiences of death visited upon our families by COVID-19.

COVID-19 as Magical Mirror

Having reached this point in the course, I was able to return to Victor Turner's (1974) concept of *liminoid*, introduced earlier in our discussion of liminality, yet I had had difficulty getting students to grasp the difference and its significance. Both concepts point to states of betwixt-and-betweenness but apply to very different social-structural conditions. Rites of passage within the context of mortuary praxis are structured, scripted, schematized, not only representing but also producing experiences of liminality for status-change purposes. Students readily drew upon the terminology of liminality in their research projects and discussions of them, but it was only at this point that I was able to clarify the critical difference between liminal and liminoid. They were invoking liminality to describe the in-between, topsy-turvy, surreal experience of #Coronachaos, yet this was hardly structured or controlled; on the contrary, it was the sort of open, floating, unintentional experience of "liminality" for which Turner coined the concept of liminoid to differentiate it from structured forms of socially controlled betwixt-and-betweenness. And once students apprehended the contrast in this context, the light-bulb went on—another pedagogical win courtesy of COVID-19. I noted this is essentially like modern life more generally: fluid and open, constantly morphing and changing and inherently unstable, premised upon capitalism's destabilizing logics of endless growth and creative destruction. The advent of COVID-19 and ensuing #Coronachaos only dramatized the situation and raised the stakes of the game.

Yet what about COVID19 in the first instance? The tiny inert piece of RNA now known as the "novel" coronavirus was in fact SARS2, hailing from a family of already-known respiratory coronaviruses. SARS1 (Severe Acute Respiratory Syndrome) materialized in 2002 and wreaked havoc for several years, which is why many Asians already wore face-masks or were primed to quickly don them. Like the others, COVID19 is a *zoonotic* disease that moved from a non-human animal host—likely bats, and possibly via another intermediary such as the pangolin—as a result of *Anthropogenic* industrialization, deforestation, and urbanization bringing humans and animals who previously had little-to-no interaction into contact (Shah 2020; Quammen 2022). This suggests that a particular bat coronavirus underwent a "spillover event" at some point in 2019 in central China, making Wuhan the original epicenter of a disease that spread quickly and wrought epic havoc throughout the world. Thus, the COVID-19 pandemic must be seen for what it is: a plague of modernity on an increasingly defiant Earth, the latest form of catastrophic convergence in the world's new geography of violence

(Parenti 2011; Hamilton 2017; Wallace-Wells 2019). Indeed, COVID-19 and #Coronachaos are manifestations of human activity in what is now called the *Anthropocene*, the geological epoch in which humans have become full-scale planet-shapers and hijacked the climate, perhaps—some contemplate—even gaining the capacity to end Nature itself (Kolbert 2014, 2021; Ellis 2018).

Like death itself, the pandemic is a magical mirror into which we could have peered and better seen our own epic liminoid late-modern-industrial Anthropogenic predicament reflected back to us—but alas, this was not to be. Yet as critics point out, it is not just any human activity or all humans that brought us the age now dubbed the Anthropocene; it is the outcome of a cultural system that organizes our political economies, our world, even ourselves. That system is *capitalism*; it has a history and operates according to specific logics, ideals, values, assumptions, rationalizations, sacrifices, and casualties. It has produced a complex and unruly spectrum of technologies, patterns of land usage, agricultural and dietary habits, productive and reproductive practices, consumption patterns, political systems, structures of financialization and indebtedness, design strategies, transportation and mobilities, digitalization, and media ecologies that increasingly subject the world to the wrath of capital. Indeed, our world is characterized by shrinking economies, savage sorting, growing expulsions, predatory financialization, and the deadening of land and water of astonishing complexity and brutality on a global scale (Sassen 2014; Hudson 2015).

Thus, some critics advocate reconceptualizing the Anthropocene as the Capitalocene, since it is not generic humanity but in fact a particular cultural system puppeteered by a changing transnational corporate oligarchy—engineered, rehearsed, and perfected within the context of colonialism—that has ushered us awkwardly into the "Anthropocene" (Moore 2016; Yusoff 2018). If we do not see what is really happening and radically change course vis-à-vis not just COVID-19 but the tip of the- iceberg it represents, we acquiesce to heading even more deeply into the corporatist-neofascist state capitalism telescoped into the future by our now even more deeply technologized present (Blakeley 2020). The climate crisis and #Coronachaos are both Anthropogenic-Capitalocenic and only a fundamental transformation of capitalism's ravenous appetite, along with industrial modernity's contempt for the natural world, will enable us to change course (Malm 2020). The pandemic represents not just pathogenic illness but social disease and moral catastrophe. Toby Miller (2021) has articulated a COVID-19 Charter identifying the steps necessary for reforming public policies and mending the inequalities and vulnerabilities that the pandemic brought into view.

#Coronachaos reveals how many of us lack pandemic literacy, with the stakes raised even higher as a problem of Anthropocene literacy as well. Yet epidemics have long shaped human affairs in profound ways. The smallpox plagues of the eastern Mediterranean in the mid-2nd–3rd centuries killed a quarter to a third of the population in the Roman Empire and triggered transformations in religious culture, leading to the expansion of Christianity and setting it on course to become the dominant religion of the empire. Several centuries later, the Justinian plague of 542–755 CE killed a quarter to half of the population in the Western Roman Empire, crippling the economy and triggering a crisis that exhausted state revenues and hobbled the imperial military, bringing about the fall of Rome. This plague also devasted the Persian Sassanid Empire, opening up new opportunities for expansion of the Islamic Rashidun Caliphate out of Arabia, not only conquering Persia but also overtaking parts of the Roman Empire in the Levant, the Caucasus, and northern Africa. The time-released effects of this trio of competing civilizations brought about the dissolution of European slavery systems and catalyzed the evolution of feudalism. Then six hundred years later, the Bubonic plague—which appeared in 1347 and burned itself out by the early 1350s—killed between a third and a half of the total European population, the socioeconomic repercussions of which signaled the end of feudalism, inspired agricultural technological innovations, accelerated processes of townification, and growing middle classes based on commerce, enterprise, and trade, also inaugurating the Renaissance. All of which in turn set the stage for the rise of capitalism and colonialism, forging new trans-Atlantic interconnections, an epic consequence of which was the unleashing of a series of epidemics among Indigenous populations throughout the Americas, undermining native life, livelihood, infrastructure and resilience, violently clearing space for the plantation machine premised upon the enslavement of sub-Saharan Africans, and conjuring the modern world-system as we know it.

How utterly humbling to think of history being conditioned so consequentially by epidemics. COVID-19 mortality rates are massive but pale in comparison with those of earlier plagues, yet perhaps numbers do not entirely matter in a pandemic of such epic, globally interconnected proportions. #Coronachaos accelerated changes already underway as well as ushered in new, unforeseen ones that are only just now unfolding and for which we do not yet have the benefit of hindsight. Will it further dissolve already-wavering faith in liberal democracy? Will it accelerate already-ongoing geopolitical shifts in the balance of power between the West and China? Will it unravel established patterns and practices of work, transportation, residence, and intimacy (Latham 2020)? The recent scourges of HIV and Ebola are zoonotic and therefore Anthropogenic in causal, epidemiological, and infrastructural dimensions. But now COVID-19 adds fuel to the fire as the latest zoonotic disease that is not only Anthropogenic as well, but in this instance also full-scale Capitalocenic in that it manifests blowback from fossil fuel-addicted industrial civilization relayed and amplified by modern globality at-large.

#Coronachaos has incited all sorts of reactions and responses, as we have already sampled in terms of my own personal and pedagogical experiences as well as the research findings and insights of my students. We are told that there is a spectacular "return of death" that has also been paradoxically reinvisibilized in line with enduring dominant modernist conceits and investments (Jacobsen and Petersen 2020). A new smartphone app called Replika provided interactive fictional digital companions—chatbot "friends"—that helped some people feel more connected and less lonely (Metz 2020). A radical Black religious studies scholar decided to stop teaching his course on "#BlackLivesMatter and Religion" since the new deathscape undermined the strategy and significance of his previous pedagogy (Gray 2021). New multiethnic "grief circles" formed in the Pacific Northwest USA in order to create space for solidarity and healing in the face of relentless crises, from fires to police brutality to COVID-19 (Short 2021). Folks in the Kambia region of northwestern Sierra Leone responded to the threat posed by the pandemic with a series of proactive community-consolidating moves and socioeconomic reconfigurations, both protecting public health and invigorating local livelihoods and social relations (Toulmin and Soulé 2021). The list goes on and on. The pandemic has also forced a digital reckoning, spawning a hybrid online-offline notion of presence as the norm going forward (Collins et al. 2021).

Meanwhile, in terms of mortuary praxis, and perhaps unsurprisingly, industrial cremation—a product of the West's Mortuary Enlightenment (Laqueur 2015)—is on the rise. Burning the dead is an apt method of corpse disposal in our liminoid age of alienation, anomie, and movement, as well as the intensifying dialectics of state and anti-state violence in and through the pandemic, premised upon an awesome harnessing of the power of fire fueled by addiction to coal, oil, and natural gas. After all, one of the alternative contenders for the Anthropocene—one promoted more by archeologists with the longer-term view—is the *Pyrocene*, which sees the arc climaxing in a hijacked contemporary climate and Earth-system destabilization as having in fact originated since at least 400,000 years ago when *Homo sapiens* domesticated fire and redirected it for their own uses. Of course, scale matters, and then is not now, but there is an elemental thread of continuity here. We know that an unintended consequence of domesticating fire was that more foodstuffs became available and a significant portion of the work of digestion was able to be performed before ingestion, thereby lessening the physiological demands of the digestive system with further unintended consequence of shifting Homo's metabolic center of gravity toward the brain—now cue the story about the human capacity for symbolic cognition and the evolution of culture.

Our near future promises to be every bit as savage as our recent past, perhaps likely even more. Roy Scranton (2015) argues that the industrial civilization which globalized and took over the world is already dying, whether one likes it or not. Ours is an unsustainable sociocultural system that cannot hold. We must learn to die culturally and existentially in the Anthropocene in order to make the most of the transition already under way. "How do we stop ourselves from fulfilling our fates as suicidally productive drones in a carbon-addicted hive, destroying ourselves in some kind of psychopathic colony collapse disorder?" (pp. 85–86) Yet nothing lasts forever. Robert Kelly (2016) sees humans as having undergone a series of radical, cumulatively synergistic transformations as a species that he calls our *beginnings*: the advent of technology more than two million years ago, the evolution of full-scale culture and language premised upon the capacity for symbolic cognition within the last couple hundred thousand years, the invention of agriculture ten to twelve thousand years ago, and the dawning of the state six to eight thousand years ago. Now we are on the threshold of another new beginning, or perhaps we have already stumbled further down the path than we realize. Humans excel at solving problems, and evolution has always been remaking us. But our latest beginning is different from the earlier ones: we now have the capacity in terms of scope and scale to change the world itself, and we have the knowledge of what we are doing as well as history to educate ourselves. We are in charge of evolution for the first time, and the future is to a very significant extent our *own* making, whether we like it or not, and whether we are up to the task or not. Pandemic literacy is death literacy is Anthropocene literacy.

Bibliography

Blakeley, Grace, *The Corona Crash: How the Pandemic Will Change Capitalism*, London: Verso, 2020.

Bloomfield, Kijan, Pandemics and the Meaning of Black Religion, *Immanent Frame* 11 (February 2021): https://tif.ssrc.org/2021/02/11/pandemics-and-the-meaning-of-black-religion/.

Collins, Samuel, Matthew Durington, and Harjant Gill, The Uncertain Present and the Multimodal Future, *American Anthropologist* 123, 1 (2021):191–193.

Ellis, Erle, *Anthropocene: A Very Short Introduction*, Oxford: Oxford University Press, 2018.

Felter, Claire, Lindsy Maizland, and Sabine Baumgartner, The Coronavirus Funeral: How the World Has Learned to Grieve in a Pandemic, *Council on Foreign Relations* (19 May 2020): https://www.cfr.org/article/coronavirus-funeral-how-world-has-learned-grieve-pandemic.

Fingarette, Herbert, *Death: Philosophical Reflections*, Chicago: Open Court Press, 1996.

Frayer, Lauren, Daniel Estrin, and Jane Arraf, Coronavirus is Changing the Rituals of Death for Many Religions, *National Public Radio* (7 April 2020): https://www.npr.org/sections/goatsandsoda/2020/04/07/828317535/coronavirus-is-changing-the-rituals-of-death-for-many-religions.

Gray, Biko Mandela, A Theodicy of the Unliving, or, Why I Won't Teach My Black Lives Matter Class Anymore, *The Immanent Frame* (7 January 2021): https://tif.ssrc.org/2021/01/07/a-theodicy-of-the-unliving/.

Hamilton, Clive, *Defiant Earth: The Fate of Humans in the Anthropocene*, Cambridge: Polity, 2017.

Hudson, Michael, *Killing the Host: How Financial Parasites and Debt Destroy the Global Economy*, Blaufelden: Institute for the Study of Long-Term Economic Trends (ISLET)-Verlag Press, 2015.

Jacobsen, Michael Hviid and Anders Petersen, The Return of Death in Times of Uncertainty: A Sketchy Diagnosis of Death in the Contemporary "Corona Crisis," *Social Sciences* 9, 8 (2020): https://www.mdpi.com/2076-0760/9/8/131.
Kelly, Robert L., *The Fifth Beginning: What Six Million Years of Human History Can Tell Us About Our Future*, Berkeley: University of California Press, 2016.
Klineberg, Stephen, *Prophetic City: Houston on the Cusp of a Changing America*, New York: Simon and Schuster, 2020.
Kolbert, Elizabeth, *The Sixth Extinction: An Unnatural History*, New York: Picador, 2014.
Kolbert, Elizabeth, *Under a White Sky: The Nature of the Future*, New York: Crown, 2021.
Laqueur, Thomas W., *The Work of the Dead: A Cultural History of Mortal Remains*, Princeton: Princeton University Press, 2015.
Latham, Andrew, How Three Prior Pandemics Triggered Massive Societal Shifts, *The Conversation* (1 October 2020): https://theconversation.com/how-3-prior-pandemics-triggered-massive-societal-shifts-146467.
Malm, Andreas, *Corona, Climate, Chronic Emergency: War Communism in the Twenty-First Century*, London: Verso, 2020.
McNeal, Keith E., Death and the Problem of Orthopraxy in Caribbean Hinduism: Reconsidering the Politics and Poetics of Indo-Trinidadian Mortuary Ritual, in *Passages and Afterworlds: Anthropological Perspectives on Death in the Caribbean*, edited by Maarit Forde and Yanique Hume, Durham: Duke University Press, 2018, 199–224.
McNeal, Keith E., Cremating the Body Politic: Mapping the Materiality of the Indo-Caribbean Mortuary Ritual Corpus, in *Folk Religions Reconsidered*, edited by Sravana Borkataky-Varma and Aaron Ullrey, New York: Routledge, 2023, 204–227.
Metz, Cade, Riding Out Quarantine with a Chatbot Friend: "I Feel Very Connected," *New York Times* (16 June 2020): https://www.nytimes.com/2020/06/16/technology/chatbots-quarantine-coronavirus.html.
Miller, Toby, *A COVID Charter, A Better World*, New Brunswick: Rutgers University Press, 2021.
Moore, Jason (ed.), *Anthropocene or Capitalocene? Nature, History, and the Crisis of Capitalism*, Oakland: PM Press, 2016.
Mural, Agência, During the COVID-19 Pandemic, Brazilian Gravediggers Face Increased Prejudice (9 September 2020), *Global Voices*: https://globalvoices.org/2020/09/09/during-the-covid-19-pandemic-brazilian-gravediggers-face-increased-prejudice/.
Ngade, Ivo, What a "Safe and Dignified" Burial Means During a Pandemic, *Sapiens* (14 January 2021): https://www.sapiens.org/culture/body-snatching-covid-19/.
Parenti, Christian, *Tropic of Chaos: Climate Change and the New Geography of Violence*, New York: Nation Books, 2011.
Public Broadcasting System, Covering Coronavirus: Life and Death in the Bronx. PBS Frontline (2020): https://www.pbs.org/wgbh/frontline/podcast/dispatch/covering-coronavirus-life-death-in-the-bronx/.
Quammen, David, *Breathless: The Scientific Race to Defeat a Deadly Virus*, New York: Simon and Schuster, 2022.
Sassen, Saskia, *Expulsions: Brutality and Complexity in the Global Economy*, Cambridge: Belknap Harvard, 2014.
Schneider-Mayerson, Matthew and Brent Ryan Bellamy (eds.), *An Ecotopian Lexicon*, Minneapolis: University of Minnesota Press, 2019.

Scranton, Roy, *Learning to Die in the Anthropocene*, San Francisco: City Light Books, 2015.
Shah, Sonia, It's Time to Tell a New Story about Coronavirus—Our Lives Depend On It, *Nation* (14 July 2020): https://www.thenation.com/article/society/pandemic-definition-covid/.
Short, April, Promoting Community Healing by Making Spaces for Grief, *LAProgressive* (March 2021): https://www.laprogressive.com/racism/promoting-community-healing.
Toulmin, Camilla and Folashadé Soulé, COVID-19 Has Helped People Understand the Vital Connection between Energy and Health, *Institute for Economic Thinking* (22 June 2021): https://www.ineteconomics.org/perspectives/blog/kandeh-yumkella-covid-19-has-helped-people-understand-the-vital-connection-between-energy-and-health.
Turner, Victor, Liminal and Liminoid in Play, Flow, and Ritual: An Essay in Comparative Symbology, *Rice University Studies* 60, 3 (1974): https://scholarship.rice.edu/handle/1911/63159.
Wallace-Wells, David, *The Uninhabitable Earth: Life After Warming*, New York: Tim Duggan Books, 2019.
Yusoff, Kathryn, *A Billion Black Anthropocenes or None*, Minneapolis: University of Minnesota Press, 2018.

Index

Note: Page numbers followed by "n" refer to end notes.